NEUROLOGIC

Commissioning Editor: Rita Demetriou-Swanwick
Development Editor: Veronika Watkins
Project Manager: Glenys Norquay
Designer/Design Direction: Stewart Larking
Illustration Manager: Merlyn Harvey
Illustrator: Graeme Chambers

NEUROLOGICAL ASSESSMENT
A Clinician's Guide

Karen J. Jones MSc SRP

Cardiff University, Heath Park, Cardiff, UK

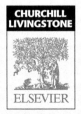

Edinburgh London New York Oxford Philadelphia
St Louis Sydney Toronto 2011

CHURCHILL
LIVINGSTONE
ELSEVIER

ISBN 978-0-7020-4052-8

Published 2014
Reprinted 2014, 2015, 2016

British Library Cataloguing in Publication Data
A catalogue record for this book is available from the British Library

Library of Congress Cataloging in Publication Data
A catalog record for this book is available from the Library of Congress

Notices
Knowledge and best practice in this field are constantly changing. As new research and experience broaden our understanding, changes in research methods, professional practices, or medical treatment may become necessary.

Practitioners and researchers must always rely on their own experience and knowledge in evaluating and using any information, methods, compounds, or experiments described herein. In using such information or methods they should be mindful of their own safety and the safety of others, including parties for whom they have a professional responsibility.

With respect to any drug or pharmaceutical products identified, readers are advised to check the most current information provided (i) on procedures featured or (ii) by the manufacturer of each product to be administered, to verify the recommended dose or formula, the method and duration of administration, and contraindications. It is the responsibility of practitioners, relying on their own experience and knowledge of their patients, to make diagnoses, to determine dosages and the best treatment for each individual patient, and to take all appropriate safety precautions.

To the fullest extent of the law, neither the Publisher nor the authors, contributors, or editors, assume any liability for any injury and/or damage to persons or property as a matter of products liability, negligence or otherwise, or from any use or operation of any methods, products, instructions, or ideas contained in the material herein.

Contents

Acknowledgements

Primarily, I wish to acknowledge the valuable guidance and support from Mrs Hilary Lipscombe who reviewed my work and acted as a consultant throughout the process. I would also like to thank Cardiff University Physiotherapy Department for supporting this project as a scholarly activity.

Special thanks to Trevor Baker for his much needed assistance in producing photographic evidence for the book and to Len Vanstone and Tim Sharp, who consented to be involved as subjects.

Lastly, I would like to take this opportunity to recognize the patience and support that is offered without question by my family and friends when life becomes a challenge.

Introduction

This book is part of *The Physiotherapist's Toolbox* series and there-fore aimed at the undergraduate student and recently qualified therapists.

AIM

The primary aim of this book is to provide the inexperienced therapist with a guide to carrying out an assessment with a neu-rologically impaired patient. From this level of assessment, safe clinical judgements can be made. These skills and knowledge combined with further clinical experience, peer support and post-graduate education will provide the stepping stones necessary for continuing development in clinical reasoning with this patient population and support the therapist's overall professional development.

CONTENT

The book is divided into three sections:

Section 1   Pathology (key facts)
Section 2   Functional Neuroanatomy
Section 3   Clinical Assessment.

The Pathology and Functional Neuroanatomy sections are aimed at providing the basic working knowledge that is most relevant to clinical practice and are therefore not exhaustive. The Clinical Assessment section begins with an introduction to assessment based on the World Health Organization's publication *Interna-tional Classification of Functioning, Disability and Health (ICF)* (2001). This is followed by general guidance through the assessment process, problem list identification, goal setting and documentation. The subjective and objective assessments are then discussed in some detail before individual chapters are used to highlight a range of clinical assessment tools. For each clinical tool, there is a description of what the procedure is assessing, why it needs to be assessed and finally a step-by-step guide to how the assessment is carried out. Photographs are inserted where relevant, to enhance the experience and provide visual cues to aid interpretation of the text. Throughout the assessment sections, additional boxes are included, highlighting any Clinical hints and tips and Cautions for the therapist to be aware of. At the end of each section is an example of how to record the findings, a brief discussion on what the findings mean (analysis) and a list of suggested outcome measures.

STRUCTURE OF THE TEXT

The three sections are sub-divided into chapters, the numbers of which run consecutively throughout the book:

Section 1	Pathology (key facts)	Chapters 1–5
Section 2	Functional Neuroanatomy	Chapters 6–15
Section 3	Assessment	Chapters 16–34.

At the start of each section is a leaf of card allowing quick and easy access to the relevant section. The section card also identifies the page numbers relating to each chapter contained within that section.

USE OF THIS TEXT

All chapters across the three sections are interlinked by a cross-referencing system, the aim of which is to guide learning and supplement understanding. The cross-referencing system within the text identifies the section number (1, 2 or 3) and the chapter number (1–34). This is abbreviated as (S••.••). This code relates to a chapter that will provide more information on the subject identified in the text. For example in the text:

'... This receptive field may be altered as a result of pathology when it can contribute to the experience of pain (S3.29) ...'

In this example, the reader is being directed to Section 3, Chapter 29, which will provide more information on pain.

The most efficient way to find this associated chapter is to:

- Go to the section card of the identified section (e.g. Section 3)
- On the section card find the chapter number (e.g. 29) and note the specific page numbers for that chapter.

The content and structure of this text can be utilized in various ways:

- The individual sections can be used as a reference text to support the development of a clinically relevant knowledge base.
- The three sections can be used to guide clinical reasoning by using the cross-referencing system to move easily between relevant information. For example, the Pathology section (key facts) defines five common neurological conditions. Each condition is cross-referenced to any relevant functional neuroanatomy and ultimately identifies the presenting signs and symptoms which are then linked to the relevant assessment tool.
- The Clinical Assessment section can also be used in isolation as a guide to clinical practice.

Karen J. Jones
2011

SECTION 1
PATHOLOGY (KEY FACTS)

PATHOLOGY (KEY FACTS)

1

INTRODUCTION

The key facts related to five pathologies are set out in the following format:

DEFINITION

A brief definition of the condition.

EPIDEMIOLOGY

This is the study of factors affecting the health and illness of populations. Common populations affected by the condition will be highlighted here.

AETIOLOGY

This is the study of causation. Where the cause of the presenting condition is known or hypothesized this will be identified.

PATHOLOGY

This is the study and diagnosis of the disease process. The pathological process underlying the condition will be explained in this section.

SIGNS AND SYMPTOMS

A *sign* is an objective indication of some medical fact or quality that may be detected by a therapist during a physical examination of a patient.

A *symptom* is a departure from normal function or feeling which is noticed by a patient, indicating the presence of disease or abnormality. A symptom is therefore subjective.

Cerebrovascular accident

DEFINITION

Cerebrovascular accident (CVA) is a clinical syndrome, of presumed vascular origin, typified by rapidly developing signs of focal or global disturbance of cerebral functions lasting more than 24 hours or leading to death (WHO 1978). If the symptoms of the lesion last less than 24 hours, the terms 'transient ischaemic attack' (TIA) or 'mini stroke' are used.

EPIDEMIOLOGY

PREVALENCE

The National UK Audit Office (DH 2006) reported that around 110000 people suffer a stroke each year, at an overall cost to the economy of around £7 billion.

AGE

Although stroke is often deemed an older person's disease, one in four people are under 65; one in ten are under 55 and 1000 people under 30 have a stroke every year.

GENDER

In the population of those aged under 75, men are at greater risk of a stroke than women.

AETIOLOGY

ISCHAEMIA (80% OF STROKES)

Damage occurs as a result of a blockage of the arteries supplying the brain (S2.8). The most common causes are thrombosis formation or emboli. A *thrombus* is the formation of a blood clot inside an intact blood vessel which obstructs the flow of blood. This can occur in large vessels such as the **internal carotid** arteries, **vertebral** arteries and those that form the circle of Willis (S2.8) or in small deeper vessels when it is termed a lacunar stroke. An *embolus* occurs when an object (the embolus) migrates from one part of the **body** (through the **circulation**) and causes the blockage of a **blood vessel** in the brain. The main sources of an embolus are a thrombus, fat droplets (following a bone fracture) or air bubbles (cardiac artery bypass graft surgery (CABG), decompression sickness, or intravenous therapy).

HAEMORRHAGE (20% OF STROKES)

Damage occurs as a result of a bleed from the circulatory system of the brain. Classification is made by location.

INTRACRANIAL HAEMORRHAGE

Intra-axial

This involves bleeding inside the brain but outside the tissue. For example, an *intraventricular haemorrhage* which occurs into the ventricles (S2.8) following moderate to severe traumatic brain injuries and is usually associated with other extensive trauma.

Extra-axial

This involves bleeding inside the skull but outside of the brain, that is between the meninges (S2.8). For example:

Epidural haematoma (EDH): A bleed between the dura mater and the skull usually caused by trauma (commonly

acceleration–deceleration), although spontaneous haemorrhage is known to occur.

Subdural haematoma (SDH): A bleed within the subdural space
often caused by head injury, when fast changing velocities
within the skull may stretch and tear small bridging veins across
the subdural space (S2.8).

Subarachnoid haemorrhage (SAH): A bleed into the subarachnoid
space (S2.8), most often caused by the rupture of an intracranial aneurysm (85%) typically at the junctions or bifurcation of
the major cerebral blood vessels. Other causes include non-
aneurysmal mid-brain haemorrhage (10%) and vascular abnormalities (arteriovenous malformation and vasculitis) (5%).

INTRACEREBRAL HAEMORRHAGE

This is a bleed that occurs within the brain tissue itself and is the
second most common cause of stroke. It may result from a ruptured aneurysm or arteriovenous malformation (AVM), invasive
brain tumour, trauma or may be spontaneous.

TRANSIENT ISCHAEMIC ATTACK (TIA)

This is thought to occur as a result of a brief interruption to the
cerebral blood supply due to thrombosis, or embolism.

PATHOLOGY

THROMBOSIS FORMATION

A thrombus is a pathological process resulting in a blood clot
forming within an intact blood vessel (Fig. 1.1). The following
conditions lead to thrombus formation. A change in the blood
vessel wall following trauma due to hypertension or the formation
of an atheroma which leads to alterations in blood flow through
the vessel. Simultaneously, a condition needs to exist that causes
a change in the blood composition, for example, hypercoagulability
disorders, smoking, hyperlipidaemia (raised lipoprotein levels),
hypercholesterolaemia or diabetes. This combination of factors
leads to aggregation of platelets to produce a platelet plug and the
activation of clotting factors, which facilitates thrombus
formation.

ATHEROMA FORMATION

An atheroma is an accumulation or swelling in the artery wall
often referred to as an atheromatous plaque and the main causal

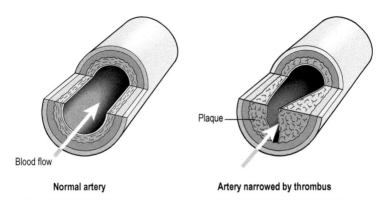

Plaque

Blood flow

Normal artery   **Artery narrowed by thrombus**

Figure 1.1 Thrombus formation in an intact blood vessel.

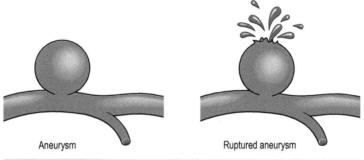

Aneurysm   Ruptured aneurysm

Figure 1.2 Aneurysm formation.

factor in thrombus formation. The disease process which results in atheroma is termed atherosclerosis. The atheroma forms between the endothelium lining and the smooth muscle wall of the artery as a result of the accumulation of white blood cells. Over time, there is a build-up which produces a lipid core surrounded by an older calcified portion.

As previously mentioned, the atheromatous plaque may lead to formation of a thrombus but it is also associated with haemorrhage resulting from aneurysm formation or plaque rupture.

ANEURYSM FORMATION

An aneurysm is a localized, blood-filled dilation of a blood vessel (Fig. 1.2) caused by disease or weakening of the vessel wall. Aneurysms most commonly occur in arteries at the base of the brain, e.g. in the circle of Willis. Aneurysm formation is probably the result of multiple factors affecting the arterial wall, however the process is probably initiated by some weakness of the vessel wall and then compounded by the blood itself bombarding the inner surface. In effect, the aneurysm becomes self-perpetuating. Risk factors for an aneurysm include diabetes, obesity, hypertension, smoking, alcoholism, and copper deficiency (which affect the elastin component of the vessel wall).

ARTERIOVENOUS MALFORMATION

Arteriovenous malformation (AVM) in the majority of cases is a congenital disorder. In the normal circulatory system, the arteries divide and sub-divide repeatedly to eventually form the capillary bed. Capillaries then successively join together, to form veins that carry blood away. In an AVM, this stepping down between the high pressure (arteries) and low pressure systems (veins) does not occur. The resultant high pressure blood flow means that the intermediate vessels become extremely fragile and prone to haemorrhage.

OUTCOME AND PROGNOSIS

The brain is highly dependent on oxygen and nutrients since it has little respiratory reserve and is completely dependent on aerobic metabolism. Brain tissue ceases to function if deprived of oxygen for more than 60–90 seconds.

Following an *ischaemic stroke,* oxygen and nutrients are depleted in the area of infarction and the production of adenosine triphosphate (ATP) fails. This sets off a series of interrelated events called an *ischaemic cascade* that can result in further secondary damage and cell death (termed 'apoptosis'), cerebral oedema and further complications related to increased intracranial pressure. Following a *haemorrhagic stroke,* the bleed acts as a space-occupying lesion within the limited capacity of the skull. Therefore the main mechanism of tissue injury may be through compression of the brain tissue. However, the loss of blood flow directly through the blood vessel and as a result of pressure leads to a loss of blood supply to the affected tissue and consequent ischaemia. The blood released from the circulatory system also appears to have a direct toxic effect on brain tissue and the vasculature.

About 10% of people who have an *ischemic stroke* recover almost all normal function and about 25% recover most of it. About 40% of people will have moderate to severe impairments requiring special care. Mortality is about 20%. About 25% of people who survive a stroke will have another stroke within 5 years.

In general, the prognosis is poor following an *intracranial* or *intracerebral haemorrhage*, with mortality rates varying between 15% and 50%. Secondary complications include hydrocephalus, raised intracranial pressure and brain herniation.

SIGNS AND SYMPTOMS

Stroke symptoms are typically of sudden onset with the presentation dependent upon the area of the brain affected. Understanding the function of the different areas of the brain (S2.7, 9, 10, 11, 12) and the blood vessels supplying them (S2.8) will give the therapist a platform by which to reason the potential clinical presentation.

The signs and symptoms presented will be a complex array of:

- Physical
- Cognitive and perceptual
- Secondary complications

PHYSICAL

Speech (S3.16)
- Dysphasia: expressive/receptive
- Dyspraxia
- Dysarthria (cranial nerves VII, IX and XII)

Swallow (S3.16)
- Dysphagia (cranial nerves IX and XII)

Sensorimotor
- Altered muscle tone (S3.21)
- Altered sensation (S3.23, 24)
- Altered reflexes (S3.22)
- Poor coordination (S3.26)
- Pain (S3.29)
- Visual deficits (S3.27)
- Poor balance (S3.32).

COGNITIVE AND PERCEPTUAL (S3.16, 17, 18, 33)
- Dyspraxia
- Inattention, neglect

- Problems with colour, depth, figure ground, form constancy, size constancy
- Problems with spatial relations for example up/down, in/out, left/right, 2D/3D
- Altered body scheme, e.g. altered midline orientation, pusher syndrome
- Agnosia: problems with recall/recognition
- Poor memory: short-term or long-term memory
- Problems with higher executive functions, e.g. planning, organization, problem solving, self-initiation, monitoring and inhibition.

SECONDARY COMPLICATIONS

- Psychosocial (S3.16): Depression, anxiety, lack of confidence, change of role, financial
- Change in postural alignment (S3.20)
- Poor core stability (S3.25)
- Altered gait (S3.19)
- Decreased muscle strength (S3.30)
- Decreased range of movement (S3.28)
- Reduced function (S3.18)
- Falls (S3.34).

REFERENCES AND FURTHER READING

Coull A, Lovett J, Rothwell P: Population based study of early risk of stroke after transient ischaemic attack or minor stroke: implications for public education and organization of services, *British Medical Journal* 328:326–328, 2004.

Department of Health: *Improving stroke services: a guide for commissioners*, 2006. Available from: www.dh.gov.uk/publications.

Furie B, Furie BC: Mechanisms of thrombus formation, *New England Journal of Medicine* 359:938–949, 2008.

Intercollegiate Stroke Working Party: *Royal College of Physicians, National Clinical Guidelines for Stroke*, ed 2, London, 2004, RCP. www.rcplondon.ac.uk.

Stroke Association: www.stroke.org.uk.

WHO: *Cerebrovascular disorders: a clinical and research classification*, Geneva, 1978, World Health Organization.

Multiple sclerosis

DEFINITIONS

Multiple sclerosis (MS) is defined as a chronic, inflammatory, demyelinating auto-immunological disease. The name multiple sclerosis refers to the scars (sclerosis), known as plaques, formed in the nervous system. There are four types of MS classified according to the course/progression of the disease process.

BENIGN MS

This subgroup is diagnosed retrospectively. These individuals show little or no disease progression.

RELAPSING REMITTING MS

This is the most common type of MS representing 80% of the people diagnosed with MS. Symptoms occur for a period of time (relapse, exacerbation) and then improve (remission), either partially or completely.

SECONDARY PROGRESSIVE MS

This type is a progression of relapsing remitting MS, when the individual shows a sustained deterioration for at least 6 months. On average, by 15 years, around two-thirds of people with relapsing remitting MS will have developed secondary progressive MS.

PRIMARY PROGRESSIVE MS

This form of MS affects around 10% of the people diagnosed. The course of the disease begins with subtle problems that worsen over time. There is no relapse remitting pattern, their MS is progressive from the beginning.

EPIDEMIOLOGY

PREVALENCE

According to government guidelines, MS is diagnosed in 3.5–6.6 people per 100 000 of the population each year in England and Wales.

AGE

MS is usually diagnosed between the ages of 20 and 50 years.

GENDER

Approximately, the ratio of women to men affected is 2:1.

GEOGRAPHY

MS occurs with much greater frequency in areas that are farther away from the equator.

AETIOLOGY

The definitive cause is unknown. However, the evidence suggests that the cause may be a combination of both genetic and environmental factors.

ENVIRONMENTAL FACTORS

Viral infection
The evidence indicates that a viral infection, produced by a widespread microbe rather than a rare pathogen, could be the origin of the disease. For example, human herpes virus, chicken pox and glandular fever.

Vitamin D deficiency
Vitamin D deficiency has been linked with a higher risk of MS. This may occur as a result of inadequate intake of the vitamin, coupled with a lack of exposure to sunlight and may explain the geographical distribution of MS in countries further away from the equator.

Other factors: environmental
Severe stress, smoking and occupational exposure to toxins may be risk factors, although the supporting evidence is weak.

GENETIC FACTORS
MS is not considered a hereditary disease. However, genetics may play a role in determining a person's susceptibility to MS.

Familial
The risk of acquiring MS is higher in relatives of a person with the disease than in the general population.

Specific genes
Differences in the human leukocyte antigen (HLA) system increase the probability of MS. These are a group of genes residing on chromosome 6 vital in immune system function. Two other genes have been shown to be linked to MS. These are the IL2RA and the IL7RA. Mutations in these receptor genes are already known to be associated with other autoimmune conditions.

PATHOLOGY

Although the initial trigger is unknown, the damage to the nervous system in MS is believed to be caused by the patient's own immune system. Lesions most commonly involve the white matter of the central nervous system in a process of demyelination. The peripheral nervous system is rarely involved.

THE PROCESS OF DEMYELINATION
The process of demyelination appears complex with the end result being damage or destruction of the oligodendrocytes in the

central nervous system by lymphocytes (white blood cells) in the immune system. This results in an inflammatory response which stimulates other immune cells, causing a number of other damaging effects such as swelling, activation of macrophages and other destructive proteins and a change in the blood–brain barrier integrity. Unlike the peripheral nervous system, damage to central nervous system is not followed by extensive regeneration as it is limited by hostile glial cells and the extracellular environment. Nevertheless, some remyelination has been found to take place in the early phases of the disease. Repeated attacks however, lead to successively fewer effective remyelinations, until a scar-like plaque (sclerosis) is built up around the damaged axons.

AXONAL LOSS

Although inflammation and demyelination has long been implicated in the pathology of MS, recent research has shown that there is also widespread loss of nerve axons in the central nervous system. The relationship between inflammation and this axonal loss is not yet fully understood, however the loss of axons is thought to be the main factor in MS progression.

OUTCOME AND PROGNOSIS

The process of demyelination results in a thinning or complete loss of myelin (Fig. 2.1) and as the disease advances, the destruction of the nerve axons. The nervous system depends crucially on the myelin sheath for insulation and support and for fast nerve conduction (S2.6) so that when the myelin is lost, the neuron no longer conducts electrical signals effectively. Of course with axon destruction, it is impossible for the neuron to conduct signals. The outcome of these processes means that communication between different parts of the central nervous system is slow, inaccurate or non-functional.

The life expectancy of an individual with MS is more or less normal. However, the mortality for older patients and those with longer disease duration is slightly higher in MS patients.

SIGNS AND SYMPTOMS

MS is an extremely variable condition. Signs and symptoms develop as the cumulative result of multiple lesions in the central nervous system. Sites of demyelination include the cerebral cortex, brain stem, spinal cord, basal ganglia, cerebellum and the cranial

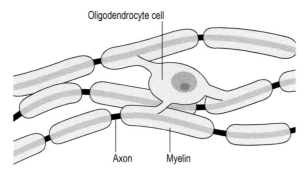

(A) Normal myelin

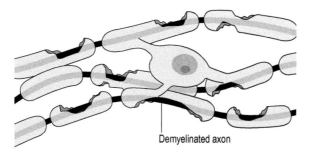

(B) Myelin partially destroyed by MS

Figure 2.1 (A) Normal myelin sheath. (B) Demyelination in multiple sclerosis.

nerves. Understanding the function of these different areas of the brain (S2.7, 9, 10, 11, 12, 13, 14, 15) will give the therapist a platform by which to reason the potential clinical presentation.

The signs and symptoms presented will be a complex array of:

- Physical
- Cognitive and perceptual
- Secondary complications

PHYSICAL

Speech (S3.16)

- Dysphasia: expressive/receptive
- Dyspraxia
- Dysarthria (cranial nerves VII, IX and XII)

Swallow (S3.16)
- Dysphagia (cranial nerves IX and XII)

Sensorimotor
- Altered muscle tone (S3.21)
- Altered sensation (S3.23)
- Altered reflexes (S3.22)
- Poor coordination (S3.26)
- Pain (S3.29)
- Visual deficits (S3.27)
- Poor balance (S3.32).

COGNITIVE AND PERCEPTUAL (S3.16, 17, 18, 33)
- Dyspraxia
- Inattention, neglect
- Problems with colour, depth, figure ground, form constancy, size constancy
- Problems spatial relations for example up/down, in/out, left/right, 2D/3D
- Altered body scheme, e.g. altered midline orientation, pusher syndrome
- Agnosia: problems with recall/recognition
- Poor memory: short-term or long-term memory
- Problems with higher executive functions, e.g. planning, organization, problem solving, self-initiation, monitoring and inhibition.

SECONDARY COMPLICATIONS
- Psychosocial (S3.16): Depression, anxiety, lack of confidence, change of role, financial
- Change in postural alignment (S3.20)
- Poor core stability (S3.25)
- Altered gait (S3.19)
- Decreased muscle strength (S3.30)
- Decreased range of movement (S3.28)
- Reduced function (S3.18)
- Falls (S3.34).

REFERENCES AND FURTHER READING

Alonso A, Jick SS, Olek MJ, et al: Incidence of multiple sclerosis in the United Kingdom: findings from a population-based cohort, *Journal of Neurology* 254:1736–1741, 2007.

Ascherio A, Munger KL: Environmental risk factors for multiple sclerosis. Part I: the role of infection, *Annals of Neurology* 61:288–299, 2007a.

Ascherio A, Munger KL: Environmental risk factors for multiple sclerosis. Part II: noninfectious factors, *Annals of Neurology* 61:504–513, 2007b.

Aulchenko YS, Hoppenbrouwers IA, Ramagopalan SV, et al: Genetic variation in the KIF1B locus influences susceptibility to multiple sclerosis, *Nature Genetics* 40:1402–1403, 2008.

Chari DM: Remyelination in multiple sclerosis, *International Review of Neurobiology* 79:589–620, 2007.

Christensen T: Human herpes viruses in MS, *International MS Journal* 14:41–47, 2007.

Compston A, Coles A: Multiple sclerosis, *Lancet* 359:1221–1231, 2002.

Filippi M, Bozzali M, Rovaris M, et al: Evidence for widespread axonal damage at the earliest clinical stage of multiple sclerosis, *Brain* 126:433–437, 2003.

Islam T, Gauderman J, Cozen W, et al: Differential twin concordance for multiple sclerosis by latitude of birthplace, *Annals of Neurology* 60:56–64, 2006.

Lünemann JD, Kamradt T, Martin R, et al: Epstein Barr virus: environmental trigger of multiple sclerosis, *Journal of Virology* 81:6777–6784, 2007.

Marrie RA: Environmental risk factors in multiple sclerosis aetiology, *Lancet: Neurology* 3:709–718, 2004.

MS Society: www.mssociety.org.

Munger KL, Levin LI, Hollis BW, et al: Serum 25-hydroxyvitamin D levels and risk of multiple sclerosis, *Journal of the American Medical Association* 296:2832–2838, 2006.

Pascual AM, Martínez-Bisbal MC, Boscá I, et al: Axonal loss is progressive and partly dissociated from lesion load in early multiple sclerosis, *Neurology* 69:63–67, 2007.

Ragonese P, Aridon P, Salemi G: Mortality in multiple sclerosis: a review, *European Journal of Neurology* 15:123–127, 2008.

Ramsaransing GS, De Keyser J: Benign course in multiple sclerosis: a review, *Acta Orthopaedica Scandinavica* 113:359–369, 2006.

Royal College of Physicians: *Multiple sclerosis: national clinical guideline for diagnosis and management in primary and secondary care,* 2004. www.rcplondon.ac.uk.

Svejgaard A: The immunogenetics of multiple sclerosis, *Immunogenetics* 60:275–286, 2008.

Waubant E: Biomarkers indicative of blood-brain barrier disruption in multiple sclerosis, *Disease Markers* 22:235–244, 2006.

Weber F, Fontaine B, Cournu-Rebeix I, et al: IL2RA and IL7RA genes confer susceptibility for multiple sclerosis in two independent European populations, *Genes and Immunity* 9:259–263, 2008.

World Health Organization: *Neurological disorders: a public health challenge,* 2006. www.who.int/mental_health/neurology/neurological_disorders_report_web.pdf.

Parkinson's disease

DEFINITION

Parkinson's disease (PD) is a progressive neurological condition, resulting from the degeneration of dopamine-producing neurons located in the substantia nigra, part of the basal ganglia (S2.11).

EPIDEMIOLOGY

PREVALENCE
The prevalence worldwide is estimated to be 4 million. In the UK, the incidence is 1 in 500 people.

ETHNIC BACKGROUND
The condition occurs in all ethnic groups.

AGE
The mean age of presentation is 65 years with peak onset between 55 and 65.

GENDER
There is a 1.8 times greater risk of PD in men than in women.

AETIOLOGY

Most people with PD are described as having idiopathic PD (having no specific known cause). The definitive cause of PD remains uncertain but is thought to result from a genetically determined vulnerability to particular environmental factors.

ENVIRONMENTAL FACTORS

Toxins
Symptoms of PD have been associated with long exposure to certain toxins/chemicals, such as pesticides and metals (e.g. manganese or iron).

Recreational drug abuse
Opioid-based recreational drugs have also been found to produce Parkinsonism type symptoms.

Head trauma
An increased risk of developing PD has been highlighted in those who have experienced a severe head injury compared with those who have never suffered a head injury. However, whether the head trauma is contributory to or a consequence of PD is still inconclusive.

GENETIC
While genetic influences may also contribute to the development of PD, it is thought to be the cause in only a small minority of cases.

PATHOLOGY

The symptoms of PD result from the loss of pigmented dopamine-secreting (dopaminergic) cells in the pars compacta region of the substantia nigra (SN). Initially, cell damage appears to occur following an excessive accumulation of iron, which is toxic to nerve cells. The outcome is oxidative stress resulting in significant damage to the proteins, lipids and DNA of the cell. A defect in the transport proteins within the cell finally leads to an abnormal accumulation of proteins (alpha-synuclein) termed a Lewy body.

OUTCOME AND PROGNOSIS

The dopaminergic neurons of the SN project to the striatum and normally modulate the activity of both the direct and indirect pathways within the basal ganglia (S2.11), having the opposite effect on each. The direct pathway facilitates the initiation and selection of the correct voluntary movement programmes to achieve a task, while the indirect pathway helps to prevent any unwanted movement programmes. In PD, the loss of dopaminergic cells in the SN means that the ability to modulate motor programme selection is lost and there is inappropriate competition between the correct and incorrect movement programmes being sent to the cortex. Consequently, a hypokinetic movement disorder presents, or in simple terms a lack of movement. As dopamine has a modulatory role (increasing or decreasing movement), a presentation of alternating background tone may also be observed (e.g. resting tremor). Also of relevance is the increased time in initiation of the long latency reflexes, which may reflect the problem with initiation of voluntary movement in PD. There are also dopamine-producing cells in three other non-motor pathways and a deficit here is thought to explain much of the neuropsychiatric pathology associated with PD. PD is both a chronic and progressive disease and although it is not considered to be fatal, the average life expectancy is generally lower than that of a healthy population.

SIGNS AND SYMPTOMS

The clinical signs of PD become evident only when about 80% of the dopamine-producing neurons are lost and may fluctuate throughout the day as a consequence of medication. When symptoms are well controlled this is termed 'on' time and when not sufficiently controlled, 'off' time (Fig. 3.1).

The signs and symptoms presented will be a combination of:

- Motor
- Sensory
- Cognitive
- Other
- Secondary complications

MOTOR

The main characteristics of the disease are often represented by the mnemonic TRAP.

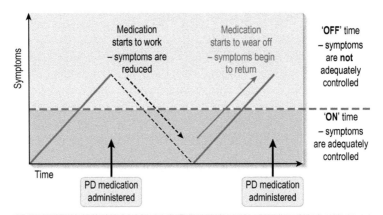

Figure 3.1 Diagrammatical representation of 'on' and 'off' times related to the medication control of Parkinson's disease (PD) symptoms.

- **Tremor (S3.18):** In the majority of patients the tremor appears when at rest and is decreased with voluntary movement. It is often referred to as pill-rolling because of its action
- **Rigidity (S3.19, 21):** Apart from affecting voluntary movement, the muscle rigidity may also limit the individual's ability to express themselves facially (masked face) or verbally (hypophonia). The lack of facial expression and weak voice often gives the wrong impression about the patient's mental state and they should be given extra time to consider and act on information given, by all concerned
- **Akinesia/bradykinesia (S3.18):** The patient becomes slower in all movements (bradykinesia) and gradually voluntary movements show a decremental loss of amplitude, and akinesia (no movement) presents. Freezing during gait is a manifestation of akinesia and often exacerbated when trying to pass through a doorway or cluttered space
- **Postural instability (S3.32):** A failure of postural reflexes results in impaired balance and may lead to falls.

SENSORY
- Pain (S3.29): Pain is common and can occur in up to 50% of people with PD. Patients may complain of sensory-type pains, which include paraesthesias, burning dysesthesias, coldness, numbness and deep aching within a nerve (neuropathic pain).

It can also be a result of musculoskeletal pain, secondary to rigidity and hypokinesia
- Impaired proprioception (S3.23).

COGNITIVE

- Depression (S3.16): This occurs in 45% of people with PD and is related to the degeneration of dopaminergic neurons in limbic and pre-frontal systems.

OTHER

- Sleep disturbances (S3.16): The causes are multifactorial but degeneration of the sleep regulation centres in the brain stem and thalamocortical pathway is implicated
- Autonomic disturbance (S3.16): Autonomic dysfunction is common in PD due to the underlying pathophysiology of the condition affecting the catecholaminergic neurons of the autonomic nervous system. Symptoms include: urinary dysfunction (40%); constipation (50%); orthostatic hypotension (a fall in systolic blood pressure of over 20 mmHg on standing) (48%); weight loss (50%) and dysphagia
- Dystonia: Abnormal, sustained, painful twisting muscle contractions are experienced by 20% of patients with PD
- Fatigue: Occurs in 50% of cases.

SECONDARY COMPLICATIONS

- Psychosocial (S3.16): Anxiety, apathy, psychosis and visual hallucinations, dementia. Change in role and financial difficulty
- Change in postural alignment (S3.20)
- Decreased muscle strength (S3.30)
- Poor core stability (S3.25)
- Altered gait (S3.19): Shuffling gait – characterized by short steps, with feet barely leaving the ground. Festinating gait – the presentation of a stooped posture, altered balance and shuffling steps results in a gait that gets progressively faster and faster, ultimately becoming unsafe
- Poor coordination (S3.26)
- Poor balance (S3.32)
- Decreased range of movement (S3.28)
- Reduced function (S3.18)
- Falls (S3.34): In the UK, two-thirds of people with PD fall at least once each year and many of them are at risk of falling again.

REFERENCES AND FURTHER READING

Ascherio A, Chen H, Weisskopf M, et al: Pesticide exposure and risk for Parkinson's disease, *Annals of Neurology* 60:197–203, 2006.

Barbeau A: Manganese and extrapyramidal disorders (a critical review and tribute to Dr George C. Cotzias), *Neurotoxicology* 5:13–35, 1984.

Bower JH, Maraganore DM, Peterson BJ, et al: Head trauma preceding PD: a case–control study, *Neurology* 60:1610–1615, 2003.

Chiueh CC, Andoh T, Lai AR, et al: Neuroprotective strategies in Parkinson's disease: protection against progressive nigral damage induced by free radicals, *Neurotoxicity Research* 2:293–310, 2000.

Di Monte DA, Lavasani M, Manning-Bog AB: Environmental factors in Parkinson's disease, *Neurotoxicology* 23:487–502, 2002.

Elbaz A, Moisan F: Update in the epidemiology of Parkinson's disease, *Current Opinion in Neurology* 24:454–460, 2008.

Goldman SM, Tanner CM, Oakes D, et al: Head injury and Parkinson's disease risk in twins, *Annals of Neurology* 60:65–72, 2006.

Hoehn M, Yahr M: Parkinsonism: onset, progression and mortality, *Neurology* 17:427–442, 1967.

Jenner P: Oxidative mechanisms in nigral cell death in Parkinson's disease, *Movement Disorders* 13:24–34, 1998.

Lepoutre A, Devos D, Blanchard-Dauphin A, et al: A specific clinical pattern of camptocormia in Parkinson's disease, *Journal of Neurology, Neurosurgery and Psychiatry* 77:1229–1234, 2006.

Lieberman A: Depression in Parkinson's disease: a review, *Acta Orthopaedica Scandinavica* 113:1–8, 2006.

Lindquist SL, Bonini NM: Parkinson's disease mechanism discovered, 2006. www.sciencemag.org.

Nambu A: A new dynamic model of the cortico-basal ganglia loop, *Progress in Brain Research* 43:461–466, 2004.

National Institute for Health and Clinical Excellence: *Parkinson's disease: diagnosis and management in primary and secondary care (Clinical guideline 35)*, 2006. www.nice.org.uk/CG035.

National Institute for Health and Clinical Excellence: *The assessment and prevention of falls in older people (Clinical guideline 21)*, 2004. www.nice.org.uk/CG021.

National Service Framework for Long-term (Neurological) Conditions. www.dh.gov.uk/longtermconditions.

The Parkinson's Disease Society: *The professional's guide to Parkinson's disease*, 2007. www.parkinsons.org.uk/PDF/PubProfessionalGuide-Nov07.pdf.

Willems A: *Rescue Consortium Katholieke Universiteit Leuven*, Belgium, 2005. Available from: www.rescueproject.org.

Xia R, Sun S, Threlkeld J: Analysis of interactive effect of stretch reflex and shortening reaction on rigidity in Parkinson's disease, *Clinical Neurophysiology* 120:1400–1407, 2009.

CHAPTER

Motor neuron disease

4

DEFINITION
Amyotrophic lateral
sclerosis (ALS)
Progressive muscular
atrophy (PMA)
Primary lateral sclerosis
(PLS)
Progressive bulbar palsy
(PBP)

EPIDEMIOLOGY
Prevalence
Age
Gender

AETIOLOGY
Familial MND
SOD1 (superoxide
dismutase1)
Other genes
Sporadic MND

PATHOLOGY
Cellular mechanisms
Aggregation (clumping)
Oxidative stress
Glutamate toxicity
Mitochondria failure
Transport disruption
Abnormal glial cells

OUTCOME AND PROGNOSIS

SIGNS AND SYMPTOMS
Motor
Amyotrophic lateral
sclerosis (ALS)
Progressive muscular
atrophy (PMA)
Primary lateral sclerosis
(PLS)
Progressive bulbar palsy
(PBP)
Secondary complications

DEFINITION

Motor neuron disease (MND) is a group of progressive neurode-generative diseases that attack the upper and lower motor neurons (S2.13). Although four distinct types of MND are described, there is a great deal of overlap between them.

AMYOTROPHIC LATERAL SCLEROSIS (ALS)

This is the most common form of MND affecting both upper and lower motor neurons.

PROGRESSIVE MUSCULAR ATROPHY (PMA)

This form is rare and only affects the lower motor neuron.

PRIMARY LATERAL SCLEROSIS (PLS)

This is a rare form of MND involving only the upper motor neurons and is usually of late onset (>50 years of age).

PROGRESSIVE BULBAR PALSY (PBP)

This form of MND affects about one-quarter of people diagnosed and involves both the upper and lower motor neuron related to the motor cranial nerves (IX, X, XII) (S2.10) and is usually of late onset (50–70 years of age).

EPIDEMIOLOGY

PREVALENCE

Approximately two people in every 100 000 develop MND per year.

AGE

MND can affect adults of any age but the highest incidence occurs between the ages of 50 and 70, with a peak between 55 and 60 years.

GENDER

Men are affected approximately twice as often as women.

AETIOLOGY

In 5–10% of MND cases, there is a strong family history evident, when it is termed 'familial MND'. However, in 90–95% of cases, the cause is unknown and termed 'sporadic MND'. More specifically, this is the term used for MND cases where there is no family history of the disease.

FAMILIAL MND

In this case MND is directly caused by a gene mutation passed down from parent to child. Unfortunately, researchers have been unable to identify a single gene as causal but several genes have been implicated:

SOD1 (superoxide dismutase1) (20% of all familial cases)
This is a detoxifying enzyme that normally removes free radicals/ toxins from the body. Normal motor neurons have very high concentrations of SOD1. In MND, a mutation in the gene manufacturing SOD1 results in the enzyme having an abnormal structure. It is suggested that the abnormal SOD1 enzyme produces further toxins instead of making them safe. The abnormal SOD1 also has an unstable structure causing it to fragment and stick together with other proteins and enzymes forming clumps or aggregates inside the cell. These clumps are the hallmark of all types of MND.

Other genes
ALS2 or alsin gene
ALS4 or Senataxin gene
ALS8 or VAPB gene
TDP-43 (TAR DNA binding protein): there is evidence to suggest that the TDP-43 protein might be involved in most cases of MND, even when the gene for its manufacture is not mutated. TDP-43 is known to be a regulatory protein and when mutated, abnormal proteins are manufactured causing the cell to malfunction. For some reason, the cell then becomes labelled for destruction.

SPORADIC MND
It is believed that sporadic MND is caused by a combination of many small contributory risk factors. Some of these risk factors are described below, however caution is advised because the supporting evidence is often circumstantial and conflicting.

Mechanical trauma: An individual, who experiences a serious head injury or more than one head injury, has a slightly higher risk of ALS
Diet: A diet lacking in polyunsaturated fat and vitamin E has been linked with individuals who have developed MND. Researchers believe that the two elements normally have a combined effect in protecting motor neurons from MND
Electrical trauma: There is some evidence that occupational exposure to extremely low magnetic fields may be linked to MND
Toxins: There is some evidence linking agricultural chemicals/ heavy metals and smoking with MND
High levels of exercise: Recent research has found a link with MND and professional football players. However, other factors such as mechanical trauma, exposure to toxic chemicals used on

football fields and the cocktail of performance-enhancing and sports injury-related drugs may also be contributory.

PATHOLOGY

Although the precise pathophysiology is unclear, the consensus of opinion indicates that the initial trigger for motor neuron degeneration comes from the motor neuron itself. However, the progression of the disease is controlled by the glial cells that surround and support motor neurons.

CELLULAR MECHANISMS

Within motor neurons there are a number of possible mechanisms that may result in this degeneration. These include:

Aggregation (clumping)

Atypical SOD1 molecules and TDP-43 proteins result in abnormal clumps of protein inside the motor neuron which disrupts the normal function.

Oxidative stress

In MND the antioxidant defence pathway, normally responsible for mopping up free radicals (toxic chemicals) produced by the motor neuron, may be suppressed.

Glutamate toxicity

In MND glutamate is present in high concentrations which can lead to excitotoxicity and cell death.

Mitochondria failure

The mitochondria in the motor neurons appear abnormal in MND. It is hypothesized that they are damaged by oxidative stress and glutamate toxicity.

Transport disruption

Research suggests that in MND, the transport system of the motor neuron is disrupted very early on in the disease process, leading to the cell working inefficiently.

Abnormal glial cells

In recent years, scientists have come to realize that it is not just motor neurons themselves that are involved in MND. The glial cells which normally provide the neurons with support may lose their supportive properties and can even become toxic. Some research suggests that this toxic event is the trigger for the other cell malfunctions (aggregation, modification of neurofilaments, mitochondrial failure, obstruction of cellular transport), and may be a consequence of SOD1 mutation.

OUTCOME AND PROGNOSIS

Although the pathophysiology seems unclear, the ultimate consequence of these processes is a degeneration of motor neurons which results in the presentation of muscle weakness. The clinical presentation and functional loss for the patient will depend upon which neurons are affected: the lower motor neuron, upper motor neurons or cranial nerves (motor only).

Amyotrophic lateral sclerosis: Average life expectancy is from 2–5 years from onset of symptoms

Progressive muscular atrophy: Most individuals live for 5–10 years

Primary lateral sclerosis: Life span could essentially be normal

Progressive bulbar palsy: This form is aggressive and relentless, with life expectancy being between 6 months and 3 years from onset of symptoms.

SIGNS AND SYMPTOMS

The signs and symptoms presented will be a combination of:

- Motor
- Secondary complications

MOTOR

Amyotrophic lateral sclerosis (ALS)

About 75% of patients experience their initial symptoms in the upper and lower limbs but in some of these cases, only one leg may be affected. About 25% of cases are of bulbar onset ALS and their presentation will be as for PBP.

- Muscle weakness (S3.30) and atrophy of muscles
- Spasticity (S3.21)
- Brisk reflexes and a positive Babinski sign (S3.22)

Progressive muscular atrophy (PMA)

- Muscle weakness or clumsiness of the hand
- No brisk reflexes or spasticity

Primary lateral sclerosis (PLS)
- Muscle weakness in lower limbs
- Spasticity in lower limbs

Progressive bulbar palsy (PBP)
- Dysarthria (cranial nerves VII, IX and XII) (S3.16): Slurring of speech. Nasality and loss of volume in speech are frequently the first symptoms
- Dysphagia (cranial nerves IX and XII) (S3.16): Difficulty swallowing. This may lead to an inability to protect the airway when eating/drinking and the risk of aspiration into the lungs.

SECONDARY COMPLICATIONS
- Cognitive: Although historically patients with MND were not considered to present with cognitive dysfunction, recent evidence has shown approximately 20% of those diagnosed with ALS do have deficits of higher executive function (S3.33) and personality
- Respiratory insufficiency: Common in patients with bulbar dysfunction, and at late stages with respiratory muscle weakness
- Psychosocial (S3.16): Depression, anxiety, lack of confidence, change of role, financial
- Change in postural alignment (S3.20)
- Poor core stability (S3.25)
- Altered gait (S3.19)
- Poor coordination (S3.26)
- Poor balance (S3.32)
- Decreased range of movement (S3.28)
- Reduced function (S3.18)
- Falls (S3.34).

REFERENCES AND FURTHER READING

Campbell WW: *The cranial nerves. DeJong's The neurologic examination*, London, 2005, Lippincott Williams and Wilkins.

Gotkine M, Argov Z: Clinical differentiation between primary lateral sclerosis and upper motor neuron predominant amyotrophic lateral sclerosis, *Archives of Neurology* 64:1545, 2007.

Hughes TA, Wiles CM: Neurogenic dysphagia: the role of the neurologist, *Journal of Neurology, Neurosurgery and Psychiatry* 64:569–572, 1998.

Kadekawa J: Clinicopathological study of a patient with familial amyotrophic lateral sclerosis associated with a two base pair deletion in the copper/zinc superoxide dismutase (SOD1) gene, *Acta Neuropathologica* 94:617–622, 1997.

Lapiedra RC, Moreno Lopez LA, Esparza Gomez GC: Progressive bulbar palsy: a case report diagnosed by lingual symptoms, *Journal of Oral Pathology and Medicine* 31:277–279, 2002.

Nixon H: Non neuronal cells. *17th International Symposium on ALS/MND*, 2006, Motor Neuron Disease Association. www.mndassociation.org/research.

Strong M: New clues on how TDP43 causes motor neurons to die. *19th International Symposium on ALS/MND*, 2008, Motor Neuron Disease Association. www.mndassociation.org/research.

Swash M, Desai J: Motor neuron disease: classification and nomenclature, *ALS and Other Motor Neuron Disorders* 1:105–112, 2000.

Tartaglia MC, Rowe A, Findlater K, et al: Differentiation between primary lateral sclerosis and amyotrophic lateral sclerosis: examination of symptoms and signs at disease onset and during follow-up, *Archives of Neurology* 64:232–236, 2007.

5 Guillain–Barré syndrome

DEFINITION

Guillain–Barré syndrome (GBS) is included in the wider group of peripheral polyneuropathies and is an autoimmune disease affecting the peripheral nervous system (PNS) characterized by a rapid demyelination, followed by remyelination. There are several types of GBS.

ACUTE INFLAMMATORY DEMYELINATING POLYNEUROPATHY (AIDP)

This is the most common form.

ACUTE MOTOR AXONAL NEUROPATHY (AMAN)

Also termed acute motor and sensory axonal neuropathy (AMSAN).

CHRONIC INFLAMMATORY DEMYELINATING POLYNEUROPATHY (CIDP)

As the name suggests, this involves a more chronic onset than other forms of GBS. Typically, patients with CIDP have a chronic progressive or relapsing remitting illness developing over at least 2 months but then potentially continuing for many years.

EPIDEMIOLOGY

PREVALENCE

GBS affects about one person in 40 000 each year in the UK.

AGE

It can occur at any age from infancy onwards but is slightly more common in the elderly.

GENDER

It is more common in men than in women.

AETIOLOGY

The definitive cause of GBS is uncertain, however in many cases there appears to be a prior infection, e.g. glandular fever or campylobacter. Recent surgery is also recognized as a triggering event.

PATHOLOGY

GBS is thought to consist of two subtypes, demyelinating (AIDP, CIDP) and axonal forms (AMAN, AMSAN). The pathological process is related to an autoimmune response towards the nerve tissue.

DEMYELINATION

The end result of such an autoimmune attack on the peripheral nerves is inflammation of the myelin sheath. In the peripheral nervous system, the cells that produce the myelin sheath are known as Schwann cells. Inflammatory cells invade the nerve tissue where they release cytokines which cause macrophages to attack and digest the myelin sheath.

AXONAL LOSS

Recent studies have demonstrated that approximately 80% of patients present with demyelination, but as many as 20% also present with axonal loss. Axonal degeneration is thought to occur due to the massive disruption of sodium channels at the nodes of Ranvier (S2.6).

OUTCOME AND PROGNOSIS

With widespread demyelination of the peripheral nerves, signal conduction (S2.6) is slowed or halted and therefore communication between systems becomes ineffective. The common course of the disease is ascending, beginning in the legs and often moving from distal to proximal body segments. Over 59% of patients reach *nadir* (maximum symptoms) within 2 weeks, 80% within 3 weeks and 90% within 4 weeks. A plateau period then begins, which may last 4–6 weeks but in some cases up to 1 year. The majority of patients require hospitalization and about 30% require ventilator assistance.

However, the PNS does have the ability for significant regeneration and therefore substantial functional recovery is possible. Initially Schwann cells repair the damage to the myelin sheath, however recovery dependent on axonal regeneration is much slower and there is often a greater degree of residual damage. This damage is considered to be the reason some patients are left with permanent weakness. Most of this recovery starts after the 4th week from the onset of the disease. Approximately 80% of patients have a complete recovery within a few months to a year, although minor findings may persist. About 5–10% of patients have one or more late relapses when they are classified as having CIDP. About 5–10% will be left with severe disability, with most of such cases involving severe proximal motor and sensory axonal damage. Mortality does occur in 2–3% of patients.

SIGNS AND SYMPTOMS

The signs and symptoms presented will be a combination of:

- Motor
- Sensory
- Autonomic
- Secondary complications

MOTOR

- Muscle weakness: potentially all muscles may be affected (S3.30)
- Reflexes: Patients may become hypo-reflexic or a-reflexic (S3.22)
- Cranial nerve involvement (S2.10): Frequently, the lower cranial nerves may be affected, leading to bulbar weakness
- Dysphagia: difficulty with swallowing (CN IX and XII) (S3.16)
- Dysarthria: (CN VII, IX and XII) (S3.16)
- Facial weakness: (CN VII)
- Eye movement abnormalities: (CN III, IV and VI)
- Fatigue: This is a common and disabling symptom in patients with GBS. There are different mechanisms associated with fatigue. A generalized lack of energy most pronounced in the morning, mental exhaustion and reduced muscular endurance, which is most dramatic in the acute phase of the illness.

SENSORY

- Numbness and tingling: often the initial symptoms in the extremities (S3.16,23)
- Loss of proprioception (joint position sense) (S3.23)
- Pain: common as a deep ache in weakened muscle (S3.29).

AUTONOMIC DYSFUNCTION

- Bladder dysfunction may occur in severe cases but should be transient
- Fluctuations in blood pressure, postural hypotension and cardiac arrhythmias are possible in severe cases of GBS.

SECONDARY COMPLICATIONS

- Respiratory insufficiency: Respiratory failure occurs in at least 17–30% of patients. Bulbar dysfunction, respiratory muscle weakness, and secondary insufficiency due to atelectasis or pneumonia are suggestive of its development
- Psychosocial (S3.16): Depression, anxiety, lack of confidence, change of role, financial

- Change in postural alignment (S3.20)
- Poor core stability (S3.25)
- Altered gait (S3.19)
- Poor coordination (S3.26)
- Poor balance (S3.32)
- Decreased range of movement (S3.28)
- Reduced function (S3.18)
- Falls (S3.34).

REFERENCES AND FURTHER READING

Barohn RJ, Lewis RA: *The alphabet soup of acute and chronic immune-mediated demyelinating polyneuropathies: similarities and differences,* 2005, Autumn newsletter of the GBS/CIDP Foundation International.

Food Standards Agency: 2008. www.food.gov.uk/science/sciencetopics/microbiology.

GBS/CIDP Foundation International: www.gbs-cidp.org.

Miller RG Katz JS: *Fatigue in Guillain–Barré syndrome,* 2005, Summer newsletter of the GBS/CIDP Foundation International.

National Institute for Neurological Disorders and Stroke (NINDS): www.ninds.nih.gov/disorders/gbs/gbs.htm.

Susuki K, Rusband MN: *Autoantibody-mediated disruption of sodium channel clusters in peripheral motor nerve fibers in axonal Guillain–Barré syndrome,* 2006. Summer newsletter of the GBS/CIDP Foundation International.

Yiu G, Zhigang H: Glial inhibition of CNS axon regeneration, *Nature Reviews Neuroscience* 7:617–627: 2006.

SECTION 2
FUNCTIONAL NEUROANATOMY

FUNCTIONAL NEUROANATOMY

2

INTRODUCTION

For accurate and effective clinical decision-making it is important to be clear about what is being assessed and what the findings mean. Sound clinical reasoning is therefore based in part upon an understanding of functional neuroanatomy. This section provides the reader with sufficient information by which to begin investigating the nervous system, however further reading will be necessary to gain a more in depth understanding.

These 10 chapters cover a broad spectrum of nervous system structures with the emphasis placed upon the knowledge that underpins the pathology and assessment sections. Each chapter is sub-divided into the basic anatomy of the structure followed by an overview of its function.

The regional functional neuroanatomy section may be used in isolation as a basic reference source or can be accessed via the cross-referencing system which guides the reader to the background knowledge relevant to topics that arise in the other two sections. For example, when reading about cerebrovascular accident, it would be useful to refresh the memory regarding the blood supply of the brain (S2.8) and the functions of the cerebral cortex (S2.7).

Introduction to excitable tissue

6

BASIC ANATOMY
  Neurons

FUNCTION OF A NEURON
  Resting potential
  Graded potential

Action potential
Summation
Conduction along a neuron
Synaptic transmission

BASIC ANATOMY

NEURONS

Neurons or nerve cells are the main components making up the nervous system and are termed 'an electrically excitable tissue' by virtue of their ability to conduct and transmit electrochemical signals throughout the body. There are many different specialized neurons, however a typical neuron (Fig. 6.1) would consist of:

Cell body, which houses the nucleus and organelles
Dendrites, which receive signals from other neurons and carry these signals towards the cell body
Axon, which conducts signals away from the cell body and onto other neurons. The axons of some neurons are myelinated and as a result are able to conduct signals faster due to its insulation properties. Myelination occurs as a result of non-neural cells wrapping themselves around the nerve axon at intervals along its length, interspersed by gaps called the nodes of Ranvier. In the peripheral nervous system, it is Schwann cells which are responsible for this function and in the central nervous system, it is oligodendrites (S2.7).

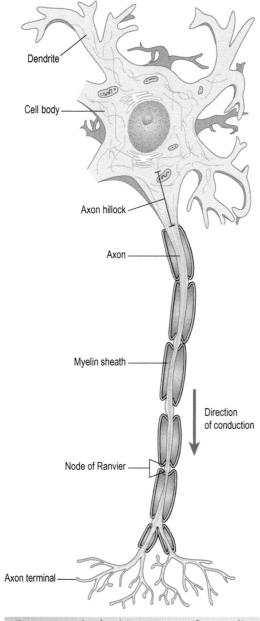

Figure 6.1 The basic structure of a myelinated neuron.

FUNCTION OF A NEURON

RESTING POTENTIAL

The neuronal cell membrane possesses a membrane potential (stored energy). This occurs because of a non-uniform distribution of ions in the intracellular (inside the cell) and extracellular (outside the cell) fluid. This distribution results due to large negative anions in the intracellular fluid and the differential permeability of ions across the membrane, most importantly sodium (Na^{2+}) and potassium (K^+). Movement of individual ions occurs according to its electrochemical gradient and continues until a balance is achieved. This balance related to all individual ions results in the inside of the neuron being *relatively* more negative than the outside of the neuron. This does not mean that the inside is negatively charged, there is just a difference between inside and outside. The typical resting potential of a neuronal cell is −70 millivolts (mV).

GRADED POTENTIAL

During a triggering event (stimulus at a sensory receptor or a signal from another neuron) there is a change in the resting membrane potential at the trigger site, which results in the depolarization of the membrane (i.e. it becomes relatively less negative). In effect, this creates a current flow in the membrane which opens voltage gated ion channels and leads to the passive movement of ions into or out of the cell. This is termed a 'graded potential'.

The magnitude of the graded potential reflects the magnitude of the triggering event. The current will flow in both directions from the active site but dies out over a short distance. Unlike an action potential, it is possible to produce further graded potentials which can build on the first.

ACTION POTENTIAL

When the cell membrane is depolarized to a threshold level (typically −50 mV) at the axon hillock (Fig. 6.1), an 'action potential' is initiated. The action potential occurs as a consequence of the high concentration of voltage gated sodium and potassium ion channels at the axon hillock. When depolarized to threshold level, these channels open on mass and initiate conduction along the axon. An action potential once initiated does not fade and therefore the signal may travel over long distances.

SUMMATION

As it is unlikely that a single graded potential will reach threshold level at the axon hillock, further graded potentials will be required. This may occur in two ways:

Spatial summation: The stimuli producing the graded potentials come from many different sources (e.g. vision, proprioception and touch).

Temporal summation: The stimuli come from the same source but at an increased frequency.

The fact that an action potential is not initiated immediately following a stimulus is beneficial, as this gives the neuron choice as to whether to respond. If the stimulus is important, the signal will be sent at the appropriate strength producing a stronger graded potential and there is more likelihood of an action potential. In simple terms, if the information is important enough, the signal will be passed on. Summation of a weaker signal gives validity to the signal before the decision is made to transmit it further. In these terms, decision-making is based at an electrochemical level.

CONDUCTION ALONG A NEURON

The ability of the signal to travel along the cell membrane is a result of the opening of sodium and potassium ion channels in response to a voltage change. In effect, a current of depolarization moves along the membrane, consecutively opening successive ion channels. Conduction of the signal can occur in two ways:

Continuous conduction: This occurs in an unmyelinated axon and each ion channel must be opened in turn for conduction to continue. This results in a slow conduction of the signal.

Saltatory conduction: This occurs in a myelinated axon. In this case, the sodium and potassium channels are concentrated within the nodes of Ranvier (Fig. 6.1) and the signal is able to jump from one node to the next making conduction much quicker. Between the nodes of Ranvier, the current travels both inside the cell (insulated by the myelin) and outside the cell (in the extracellular fluid).

SYNAPTIC TRANSMISSION

The junction between two neurons is termed a 'synapse' and represents a gap between the two neurons. In order for a signal to be passed from a pre-synaptic neuron to a post-synaptic neuron, the electric signal (the action potential) is transformed into a chemical signal (the neurotransmitter substance), which is released into the synaptic cleft and diffuses across the gap. The neurotransmitter attaches to specific ion receptors on the post-synaptic cell, which results in the opening of the ligand/chemically gated ion channels. Each synapse is highly specific in terms of the ion channels it possesses so that only movement of one particular ion occurs. The direction of ion movement is dictated by the existing chemical gradient. For example, sodium moves into the cell and potassium moves out of the cell.

Ultimately, what is produced in the post-synaptic membrane is a graded potential. Depending upon the ion channels present, the graded potential may result in:

Depolarization: This is termed 'an excitatory post-synaptic potential' or EPSP and occurs as a result of sodium (Na^+) entering the cell. The membrane potential therefore becomes less negative and hence nearer to the threshold for initiating an action potential. These are often referred to as 'excitatory synapses'.

Hyperpolarization: This is referred to as an 'inhibitory post-synaptic potential' or IPSP and occurs when either chloride ions (Cl^-) enter or potassium (K^+) ions leave the cell. In either case, the membrane potential becomes more negative and hence further from threshold potential. Therefore an action potential is less likely to occur. These are often referred to as 'inhibitory synapses'.

REFERENCES AND FURTHER READING

Sherwood L: *Human physiology: from cells to systems*, ed 6, Australia, 2007, Thomson Brooks/Coles.

Tortora GJ, Derrickson B: *Essentials of anatomy and physiology*, ed 8, Hoboken, 2010, John Wiley and Sons.

7

The cerebral cortex

BASIC ANATOMY

The cerebral cortex or cerebrum is a structure within the brain that plays a key role in all that we do, think and feel.

HEMISPHERES

The brain is divided into two halves or hemispheres, which are divided into four lobes (frontal, parietal, temporal and occipital) (Fig. 7.1). The left and right hemispheres are connected by the corpus callosum (Fig. 7.2), which facilitates communication between the two sides of the brain. The limbic system, sometimes referred to as a 5th lobe, forms the inner border of the cortex and is made up of several different structures scattered throughout the four lobes.

GREY/WHITE MATTER

The outermost layer of the cerebral cortex is termed the 'grey matter' (Fig. 7.2) and is primarily composed of the cell bodies of neurons (S2.6). The grey matter is an expansive sheet, approximately 2–4 mm (0.08–0.16 inches) thick, which is intricately folded to form grooves termed 'sulci' and raised areas termed

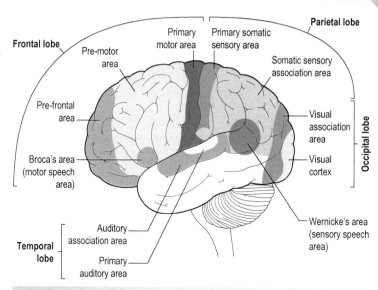

Figure 7.1 Anatomical map of the cerebral cortex – lateral surface.

'gyri' (Fig. 7.2). The compact nature of the grey matter allows closer contact between neurons and consequently faster communication. The white matter (Fig. 7.2) below is formed predominantly by the myelinated axons of the neurons (S2.6), which connect to different regions of the central nervous system.

THE INTERNAL CAPSULE

The internal capsule lies superiorly to the thalamus (S2.9) and consists of neurons passing from the thalamus to the cerebral cortex and vice versa. Between the cortex and the internal capsule, the ascending and descending neurons form the corona radiata. All afferent and efferent information is routed through the internal capsule and most sensory information enters the cerebral cortex via the thalamus.

CONNECTIONS

The left and right hemispheres of the cerebral cortex are connected by corpus callosum with each hemisphere being connected, in the main, to the contralateral side of the body. Thereby

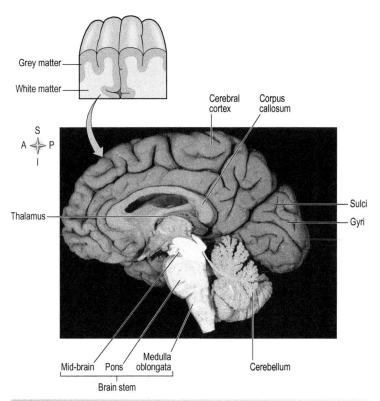

Figure 7.2 Anatomical map of the cerebral cortex – medial surface.

the left hemisphere receives information from the right side of the body and has motor control of the right side of the body. This is the result of the decussation or crossing of the ascending and descending tracts (S2.14, 15). However, there are a minority of neurons which remain ipsilateral, e.g. in the corticospinal tract (S2.14). That is, some neurons within the tracts remain on the same side of the body. This phenomenon is thought to have important implications during rehabilitation of neurologically impaired patients, especially those following stroke.

The hemispheres are richly connected to various subcortical structures such as the thalamus (Fig. 7.2) and basal ganglia, however the vast majority of connections (99%) are from one area of the cortex to another.

CELLS OF THE CEREBRAL CORTEX

Neurons

In the cerebral cortex there are two main forms of neuron – those which result in excitatory post-synaptic potentials (EPSP) and others producing inhibitory post-synaptic potentials (IPSP) (S2.6). The excitatory neurons may span several layers enabling them to pick up a wide range of information. They often have a high density of dendrites which are covered in post-synaptic sites called 'spines', further reinforcing this role. Inhibitory neurons however, tend to be in the minority (20%) and are more diverse in their characteristics. They often remain within the grey matter making short range local connections. Their role is considered to be modulation. Modulation is not necessarily a case of switching other neurons 'on' or 'off' but rather to grade or fine tune in the same way as we would use a dimmer switch for a light.

Glial cells

Glial cells, commonly called 'neuroglia' or 'glia' are non-neuronal cells which outnumber neurons by about 10 to 1. The four main functions of glial cells are to provide structural support for neurons, to supply neurons with nutrients and oxygen, to insulate one neuron from another and to destroy pathogens and remove dead neurons (Table 7.1).

Glial cells have often been considered the passive bystanders of neural transmission. However, recent studies have discovered glial cells are essential to the process. Unlike the neuron, which is generally considered incapable of mitotic division, glial cells continue cell division into adulthood.

FUNCTION OF THE CEREBRAL CORTEX

OVERVIEW

The areas responsible for encoding sensory information and commanding movement account for about one-fifth of the cerebral cortex. These areas that function to integrate information and produce a meaningful experience of the world are termed the 'association areas'.

The integration of sensory information takes place in the parietal, temporal and occipital lobes, typically in the right hemisphere. The frontal lobe or pre-frontal association area is involved in planning actions and movement, as well as abstract thought. Our language abilities are localized to the association

Table 7.1 Types of glial cells and their functions

Classification of glial cells	Glial cells	Function in brief
Microglia	Specialized macrophages	Phagocytosis to protect neurons in the CNS
Macroglia	Radial glia	In development, function as progenitor and support cells. In mature CNS only found in cerebellum (regulate synaptic plasticity) and retina (for communication with neurons)
	Ependymal cells	These create, secrete and circulate cerebrospinal fluid in the cavities of the CNS (e.g. ventricles)
	Oligodendrocytes	Produce the myelin sheath for neurons in the CNS
	Astrocytes	Anchor and regulate the blood supply to neurons. Remove excess ions and recycle neurotransmitter released during synaptic transmission. Form the building blocks of the blood–brain barrier. Able to signal each other using calcium

areas of the parietal-temporal-occipital lobes, typically in the left hemisphere.

SENSORY

The sensory areas are located in both hemispheres of the cortex in the parietal, temporal and occipital lobes and receive and process information from the sensory receptors. The parts of the cortex that receive sensory input from the thalamus are called the primary sensory areas. The senses of vision, audition and touch are served by the primary visual cortex (occipital lobe), primary auditory cortex (temporal lobe) and primary somatosensory cortex (parietal lobe). The latter receives information about the contralateral side of the body.

There is a regional specialization of function within the sensory areas. In simple terms, this means that neurons performing similar roles and therefore needing to communicate efficiently will tend to be found together. This organization gives rise to a cortical map of the sensory area known as a 'topographic map'. The somatosensory topographic map is represented by a deformed human shape and is termed the 'homunculus' (Fig. 7.3). In the homunculus, the sizes of the different body parts reflect their relative importance in terms of the density of innervations. For example, areas with lots of sensory receptors, such as the fingertips and the lips have a larger area of representation because the number of sensory neurons entering the sensory cortex is greater.

MOTOR

The motor areas are located in both hemispheres of the frontal lobe and control the contralateral side of the body; they are also arranged topographically forming a motor homunculus (Fig. 7.3). Three main areas of the cortex have been found to be important in voluntary movement:

The dorsolateral pre-frontal cortex *decides* on the voluntary movements required according to higher-order instructions, rules, and self-generated thoughts.

The supplementary motor area and pre-motor areas *select* voluntary movements from learned stored memory or motor programmes.

The primary motor cortex *executes* voluntary movement and is integrally linked with the primary somatosensory cortex.

ANATOMICAL AREAS AND THEIR FUNCTION LINKED TO ASSESSMENT

Based upon past and present research, Tables 7.2–7.6 represent a summary of the basic functions of the four main lobes and the limbic lobe. Each table also includes the terminology used to describe a dysfunction of the relevant function and the section/ chapter code linking it to an assessment tool, where appropriate. It may be useful to read these tables in conjunction with Figure 7.1, which shows the anatomical position of these areas within the lobes of the cerebral cortex.

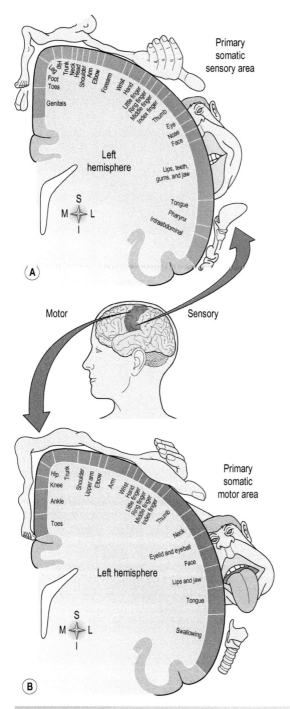

Figure 7.3 The sensory and motor homunculus.

Table 7.2 Functional localization of cerebral cortex: frontal lobe

Area	Function	Dysfunction	Assessment chapters
Primary motor cortex	Voluntary control of movement	Poor motor control during voluntary movement. Altered muscle tone	S3.16, 18, 21
Pre-motor area (PMA) (lateral pre-motor area)	The PMA is involved in the selection of movements based on external events, a sensory guidance system (e.g. visual cues) (Shima and Tanji 1998; Cunnington et al. 2002)	Dyspraxia	S3.16, 33
Supplementary motor area (SMA) (medial pre-motor area)	The SMA mediates the selection of movement from stored plans specified by internal cues (e.g. self-initiated or spontaneous movements – from memory) (Weilke et al. 2001)		
	Both implicated in the planning of motor actions		
Pre-SMA	Pre-SMA is involved in acquiring new sequences. In contrast, SMA is involved when performing a sequence already learned (Cunnington et al. 2005). Some authors believe that the full function of these areas has not yet been established (Nachev et al. 2008)		
Broca's area	Left hemisphere for expression of speech. Right hemisphere for non-verbal communication	Expressive dysphasia	S3.16
Pre-frontal cortex	Personality and behaviour (an appreciation of 'self')	Change in character, inappropriate behaviour	
	Higher executive function – problem-solving, initiation, moderation and termination of behaviour. Also linked to the basal ganglia to form a loop which regulates cognitive function	Dysexecutive syndrome	S3.16, 33

Table 7.3 Functional localization of cerebral cortex: parietal lobe

Area	Function	Dysfunction	Assessment chapters
Primary somatosensory cortex	Receives sensory information from the whole body. Homunculus representation	Altered sensation	S3.16, 23
Sensory association areas:	Integrates information from sensory areas; thoughts based on a variety of sensory inputs		
Inferior parietal lobe	The primary region governing attention. Right hemisphere mediates attention to both left and right sides of the body. Left hemisphere only the right side of body. Therefore only damage to the right hemisphere results in neglect, as left hemisphere damage can be compensated for by the intact right hemisphere (Purves et al. 2000)	Contralateral neglect: Inability to perceive and attend to objects, space or own body, despite vision, somatosensation and motor ability being intact	S3.16, 33
Visual association area	Processing of visual information for perception of motion and spatial relationships in the environment. The 'where and how' pathway	Problems with visuospatial awareness (e.g. 3-dimension/2-dimension, figure ground)	S3.16, 33

Table 7.4 Functional localization of cerebral cortex: temporal lobe

Area	Function	Dysfunction	Assessment chapters
Primary auditory cortex	Topographically arranged. Loudness, pitch and localization of basic sounds	Deafness	S3.16
Temporal association areas:	Information processed for recognition and identification of stimuli attended to	Agnosia. Acknowledge existence of a stimulus but are unable to report what it is	S3.16, 33
Right inferior temporal lobe	Face and object recognition	Prosopagnosia: unable to identify faces	
Auditory association area (superior temporal lobe)	Less organized topographically but specialized for processing complex sound, e.g. speech		
Wernicke's area (left inferior temporal lobe)	Reccgnizes spoken words and interprets meaning of speech	Receptive dysphasia	S3.16
Visual association area	Processing of visual information related to form recognition and object representation. The 'what' pathway. Storage of long-term memory	Problems with visuoperceptual awareness (e.g. form constancy)	S3.16, 33
Pyriform cortex	Main centre for processing olfactory sensations		
Insula cortex	Processes taste sensation (anterior)		

Table 7.5 Functional localization of cerebral cortex: occipital lobe

Area	Function	Dysfunction	Assessment chapters
Primary visual cortex	Topographically arranged. Determines the basic attributes of vision: light, shape, colour, size, direction. Binocular function, i.e. signals from left and right eyes are combined – allowing depth perception. Processing occurs in several areas: temporal lobe – recognition; parietal lobe – spatial relations.	Double vision (diplopia) Blindness	S3.16, 27
Visual association area	Generally respond to visual stimuli within their receptive fields but are modulated by attention and working memory. Processing occurs in other cortical areas.		

Table 7.6 Functional localization of cerebral cortex: limbic system

Area	Function	Dysfunction	Assessment chapters
Hypothalamus (temporal lobe)	Centre for coordinating autonomic (visceral) and motor (expression) components for emotional behaviour	These pathways provide the cortical control of emotion. Damage results in altered emotional behaviour. Inability to lay down new memories (hippocampus)	S3.16
Mamillary body (posterior temporal lobe)	Connects hypothalamus and cingulate cortex. Processing of recognition memory		
Cingulate gyrus (frontal and parietal lobes)	Projects to the hippocampus. Involved in motor planning and regulation of cognitive and emotional processing via its link to the basal gangia	Right hemisphere more important for the perception of emotion in others (e.g. from faces) and expression of own emotion (e.g. in speech/face). Damage leads to aprosodia (monotone speech)	
Hippocampus (medial temporal lobe)	Projects back to hypothalamus via fornix. Important in establishing new declarative memories		
Parahippocampus (surrounds hippocampus)	Important role in memory encoding and retrieval, especially of spatial memory (e.g. rooms, landscapes)	Right hemisphere associated with positive moods. Damage leads to depressed mood	
Amygdala (ant-medial temporal lobe)	Major role in giving emotional significance to a sensory experience. Achieves this via many links to pre-frontal cortex and subcortical structures (e.g. thalamus, basal ganglia, reticular formation and cranial nerves) (S2.10)	Left hemisphere associated with negative moods. Damage leads to being 'unduly cheerful' (Purves et al. 2000)	
Orbital frontal lobe	Linked to amygdala. Integrates a combination of information from vision, somatosensory, olfactory and taste sensations. Involved in the motivation to eat or not		

REFERENCES AND FURTHER READING

Burns GA, Young MP: Analysis of the connectional organization of neural systems associated with the hippocampus in rats. Philosophical Transactions of the Royal Society, Series B, *Biological Sciences* 355:55–70, 2000.

Cunnington R, Windischberger C, Deecke L, et al: The preparation and execution of self-initiated and externally-triggered movement: a study of event related fMRI, *Neuroimage* 15:373–385, 2002.

Cunnington R, Windischberger C, Moser E: Premovement activity of the presupplementary motor area and the readiness for action: studies of time-resolved event-related functional MRI, *Human Movement Science* 24:644–656, 2005.

Herrup K, Yang Y: Cell cycle regulation in the postmitotic neuron: oxymoron or new biology? *Nature Reviews Neuroscience* 8:368–378, 2007.

Nachev P, Kennard C, Husain M: Functional role of the supplementary and pre-supplementary motor areas, *Nature Reviews Neuroscience* 9:856–869, 2008.

Passingham RE, Stephan KE, Kotter R: The anatomical basis of functional localization, *Nature Reviews and Neuroscience* 38:606–616, 2002.

Purves D, Augustine GJ, Fitzpatrick D, et al: *Neuroscience*, Sunderland, 2000, Sinauer Associates.

Shima K, Tanji J: Both supplementary and presupplementary motor areas are crucial for the temporal organization of multiple movements, *Journal of Neurophysiology* 80:3247–3260, 1998.

Shipp S: Structure and function of the cerebral cortex, *Current Biology* 17 12:R443–R449, 2007.

Weilke F, Spiegel S, Boecker H, et al: Time-resolved fMRI of activation patterns in M1 and SMA during complex voluntary movement, *Journal of Neurophysiology* 85:1858–1863, 2001.

Welker W: Why does the cerebral cortex fissure and fold? A review of determinants of gyri and sulci. In Jones EG, Peters A, editors: *Cerebral Cortex, Vol 8b: Comparative structure and evolution of cerebral cortex, Part 2*, New York, 1991, Plenum Press.

Wolosker H, Dumin E, Balan L, et al: Amino acids in the brain: d-serine in neurotransmission and neurodegeneration, *The FEBS Journal* 275(14):3514–3526, 2008.

Young MP, Hilgetag CC, Scannell JW: On imputing function to structure from the behavioural effects of brain lesions. Philosophical Transactions of the Royal Society, Series B, *Biological Sciences* 355:147–161, 2000.

Meninges, ventricular system and blood supply

 MENINGES

BASIC ANATOMY

The brain and spinal cord are surrounded by three membranes termed 'meninges', which primarily protect and cushion the brain, brain stem and spinal cord.

Dura mater

This outer layer is conventionally described as two layers, however they are closely united except along certain lines where they part to surround and support large venous channels termed 'the dural venous sinuses' (Fig. 8.1). The two layers comprise:

The endosteal layer, which represents the periosteum covering the inner surface of the skull bones.
The meningeal layer, which is the dura mater proper. This is a thick, dense, strong fibrous sheet covering the brain and it is continuous with the dura mater of the brain stem and spinal cord.

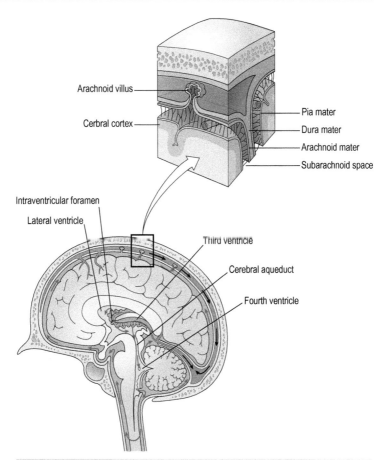

Arachnoid villus

Cerbral cortex

Pia mater

Dura mater

Arachnoid mater

Subarachnoid space

Intraventricular foramen

Lateral ventricle

Third ventricle

Cerebral aqueduct

Fourth ventricle

Figure 8.1 The ventricular system showing a dural venous sinus.

Arachnoid mater

This middle layer is a delicate web-like structure lying between the dura mater and pia mater. The space between the dura mater externally and the arachnoid mater is called the 'subdural space'. The space between the pia mater internally and the arachnoid mater is the 'subarachnoid space'. The major arteries to the brain pass through the subarachnoid space and it is also filled with cerebrospinal fluid. This space extends down the spinal cord to the level of the second sacral vertebra.

In certain areas, the arachnoid mater projects into the dural venous sinuses to form arachnoid villi or granulations (Fig. 8.1) via which cerebrospinal fluid is recycled into the venous blood system.

Pia mater

This inner layer is a very delicate impermeable vascular membrane closely covering the brain surface (Fig. 8.1).

FUNCTION OF THE MENINGES

The outermost covering, the dura mater, serves to protect the underlying nervous tissue of the central nervous system and also has a role in restricting the displacement of the brain during head movement.

The primary function of the arachnoid mater and the space enclosing the cerebrospinal fluid is to further cushion the central nervous system. The pia mater supports capillaries that enter the tissue of the cerebral hemispheres.

THE VENTRICULAR SYSTEM

BASIC ANATOMY

The ventricles are a system of spaces within the cerebral hemispheres, which produce and circulate cerebrospinal fluid around the central nervous system.

Ventricles

The ventricular system incorporates a series of interconnected spaces in the core of the brain. The largest spaces are the lateral ventricles, which are bilateral and are the site of the choroid plexus, which produce cerebrospinal fluid. The 3rd ventricle is linked to the lateral ventricles by the interventricular foramina and to the 4th ventricle by the cerebral aqueduct. The 3rd and 4th ventricles lie in midline (Fig. 8.1).

Cerebrospinal fluid

Cerebrospinal fluid (CSF) is a clear fluid produced by the choroid plexuses within the lateral ventricles. The CSF circulates through the ventricular system and ultimately enters the subarachnoid space which surrounds the cerebral cortex, cerebellum, brain stem and spinal cord down to the level of the second sacral vertebra. The CSF is recycled into the dural venous sinuses via the arachnoid villi (Fig. 8.1) and returned to the venous circulation.

FUNCTION OF THE VENTRICULAR SYSTEM

The primary role of the CSF is the removal of waste products after neuronal activity and to provide basic mechanical and immuno-

logical protection to the nervous system. Along with the meninges, the CSF also cushions the delicate central nervous system
from rubbing against the bony skull and vertebral column. The
amount of CSF within the system can be regulated in order to
maintain the correct intracranial pressure (ICP), so facilitating
cerebral blood flow. Any disruption or blocking of the flow of
CSF may result in cerebral oedema, reduced blood flow and brain
damage.

CIRCULATORY SYSTEMS OF THE BRAIN

ARTERIAL SUPPLY

Basic anatomy

Normal function of the brain's control centres is dependent upon
an adequate supply of oxygen and nutrients through a dense
network of blood vessels. The brain represents approximately 2%
of the total body weight, however it receives 20% of the resting
cardiac output. Blood is supplied by the two internal carotid arteries and the two vertebral arteries that join at the base of the brain
to form the basilar artery.

Anterior circulation   The carotid arteries and their branches are
referred to as the 'anterior circulation'. The left common carotid
artery arises from the aortic arch (Fig. 8.2). The right common
carotid arises from the innominate artery. From each common
carotid artery there are two branches:

The *external carotid*, which supplies the face, neck and
    meninges.
The *internal carotid*, which supplies the brain.

The left and right internal carotid arteries pierce the dura mater
at the base of the brain and each bifurcates to form the anterior
cerebral artery and the middle cerebral artery (Fig. 8.2).

Posterior circulation   The vertebrobasilar system is referred to as
the 'posterior circulation' (Fig. 8.2).

The vertebral arteries arise from the subclavian artery and
ascend through the transverse foramina of the cervical vertebrae
entering the skull through the foramen magnum. The vertebral
artery gives off branches to the spinal cord, the cerebellum and
to the medulla.

The two vertebral arteries join at the junction of the pons and
medulla oblongata (S2.10) to form the basilar artery, which then

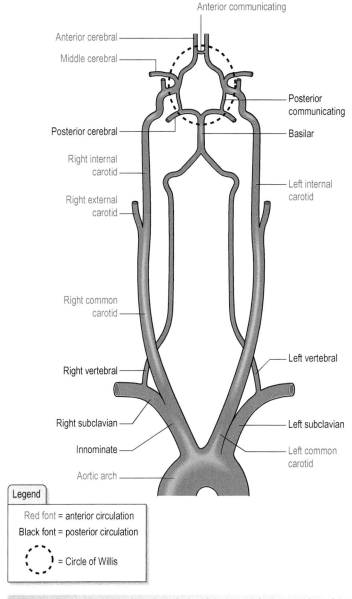

Figure 8.2 Arterial supply of the brain and the circle of Willis.

divides at the junction of the pons and mid-brain to form the two posterior cerebral arteries (Fig. 8.2). It also gives off branches to the cerebellum.

The circle of Willis   The circle of Willis (Fig. 8.2) is a polygon shaped network of blood vessels beneath the cerebral hemispheres. The two anterior cerebral arteries are connected by the anterior communicating artery and the posterior cerebral arteries are connected to the ipsilateral internal carotid arteries by the posterior communicating arteries. The six cerebral arteries, bilaterally the anterior, posterior and middle are termed end arteries.

Function of the arterial supply

The blood supply aims to meet the physiological demands of the brain cells, including neural and non neural cells. Delivering oxygen, glucose and nutrients is a high priority as these tissues have a high metabolic rate and are highly sensitive to oxygen deprivation. A compromised blood supply lasting only seconds can cause neurological symptoms and after minutes, can lead to permanent damage.

The anatomical arrangement of the circle of Willis functions to provide the main vessels supplying the brain with a safety net. The circle design means that if there is damage to one of the main vessels, the distal smaller arteries can still be supplied from the other arteries in the circle (collateral circulation). However, if damage occurs to the end arteries, there is no such collateral circulation and consequently, brain damage cannot be avoided.

Understanding the area each main artery supplies and the function of that area allows the clinician to begin predicting the potential presentation of a patient prior to assessment:

The vertebral arteries   These supply the spinal cord via the medullary arteries which join to form the anterior and posterior spinal arteries. Based upon the general arrangement of the descending tracts anteriorly and the ascending tracts posteriorly, damage to these blood vessels could result in a motor loss or sensory loss, respectively.

The basilar artery   This is formed by the two vertebral arteries. Branches from this posterior circulation supply the brain stem and cerebellum.

The anterior cerebral arteries   Bilaterally, these supply the inferior parts of the frontal lobe, the medial surface of the frontal and parietal lobes and the anterior part of the corpus callosum. Branches from the anterior cerebral artery supply the limbic system, basal ganglia and anterior limb of the internal capsule.

The middle cerebral arteries   Bilaterally, these supply large parts of the frontal, temporal and occipital lobes and the parietal lobe. Branches from the middle cerebral artery supply the basal ganglia and posterior limb of the internal capsule.

The posterior cerebral arteries   Bilaterally, these supply the inferior temporal and occipital lobes, the posterior part of the corpus callosum and the thalamus.

THE BLOOD–BRAIN BARRIER

A stable physiological environment within the brain is crucial for normal function. Neurons need to be protected from changes in this micro-environment. This is achieved by the blood–brain barrier, a specialized interface between the capillary walls and the surrounding neural tissues that restricts the passage of various chemical substances and microscopic objects such as bacteria between the blood and the neural tissue itself.

In other areas of the body, free movement of ions and molecules back and forth across the tissue boundary is permitted. However, in the brain, the endothelial cells of the capillary wall overlap and form tight junctions termed 'end feet' with astrocyte cells (S2.7) surrounding them. The astrocytes also provide them with biochemical support. Thus, there is little free movement from blood into the interstitial environment of the neural tissue. There are however, specific transporters across the barrier for critical ions and molecules such as glucose and specific amino acids.

VENOUS DRAINAGE

Basic anatomy

The venous drainage of the brain can be separated into two sub-divisions:

Superficial   The superficial system is composed of dural venous sinuses (Fig. 8.1) located on the surface of the cerebrum. The dural venous sinuses are situated between the two layers of the dura mater and lined with endothelium. They differ from other vessels in that their walls lack the characteristic layering, muscle and valves seen in other veins. Their function is to receive blood from the deep and superficial cerebral veins and cerebrospinal fluid from the subarachnoid space via the arachnoid villi and empty these components into the internal jugular vein to be returned to other organs for recycling.

Deep The deep venous drainage is primarily composed of traditional veins inside the deep structures of the brain. However, the cerebral veins are thin walled and have no valves.

At the confluence of sinuses, the superficial and deep venous drainage join and form the two internal jugular veins. In the neck, the jugular veins run parallel to the upward course of the carotid arteries and ultimately drain blood into the superior vena cava.

FUNCTION OF VENOUS DRAINAGE

The veins carry deoxygenated blood back to the heart, removing carbon dioxide, lactic acid and other metabolic products.

REFERENCES AND FURTHER READING

Sherwood L: *Human physiology: from cells to systems*, ed 6, Australia, 2007, Thomson Brooks/Coles.

Tortora GJ, Derrickson B: *Essentials of anatomy and physiology*, ed 8, Hoboken, 2010, John Wiley and Sons.

Thalamus and limbic system

BASIC ANATOMY OF THE THALAMUS

The thalamus is believed to both process and relay sensory information *selectively* to various parts of the cerebral cortex. The two thalami are prominent bulb-shaped masses about 5.7 cm in length, located on each side of the 3rd ventricle, and form the major part of the diencephalon. The thalamus is composed of a complex system of myelinated neurons separated by distinct clusters of neuron cell bodies, which form specific nuclei. Figure 9.1 shows the anatomical arrangement of the thalamus, with clusters of nuclei being divided into three main parts: anterior, medial and

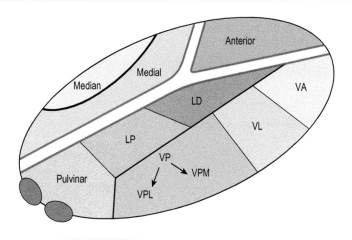

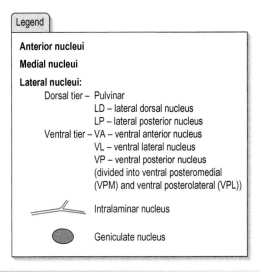

Figure 9.1 Anatomical relationship of the thalamic nuclei.

lateral, by the intralaminar nucleus. The lateral part is further sub-divided into dorsal and ventral tiers.

FUNCTION OF THE THALAMUS

Traditionally, the thalamus was considered to act as a relay station within the central nervous system subserving both sensory and motor mechanisms. However, the extent of its afferent and efferent connections with the periphery and the brain and the mass of interconnections between the thalamic nuclei implies that in addition, it has a significant role in controlling and modifying this information. More precisely, the corticothalamic system appears to synchronize the activity of thalamic and cortical neurons.

As a result of its widespread connections, damage to the thalamus may cause a range of presentations.

FUNCTION OF THE THALAMIC NUCLEI

The anterior part

This part is strongly connected to the limbic system (cingulate nucleus and hypothalamus) and is concerned with muscle tone related to our emotional state.

The medial part

Particularly the *dorsomedial nucleus* has reciprocal connections with the pre-frontal cortex in the frontal lobe, the hypothalamus and all other thalamic nuclei. Its role is the integration of all sensory, motor and visceral information entering the thalamus concerning our emotional state.

The medial and anterior parts also receive information from the spinothalamic tract (pain and temperature), which relates to the 'medial pain system' and projects to the anterior cingulate cortex. This area is consistently activated by noxious stimuli and has been associated with the affective–emotional aspect of pain.

The lateral part/dorsal tier

These nuclei connect with other thalamic nuclei and with the lobes of the cerebral cortex (with the exception of the frontal lobe) but little is known of their function.

The lateral part/ventral tier

The ventral lateral and ventral anterior nuclei are connected to the reticular formation, basal ganglia and the pre-motor cortex, hence influencing motor output from the cortex.

The ventral posterior nucleus (posterolateral and posteromedial) receive information related to taste, pain, temperature, and light touch, which is relayed through the posterior limb of the internal capsule to the primary somatosensory cortex. The 'lateral pain system' is included here and projects to the primary somatosensory cortex, related to the sensory-discriminative dimension of pain; the secondary somatosensory cortex, related to pain intensity; and to the insula for pain information processing.

Intralaminar nuclei

These nuclei receive connections from the reticular formation and are involved in regulating the level of consciousness and arousal. Neurons also project on to wide areas of the cortex and the basal ganglia.

Paramedian nuclei

These nuclei also receive input from the reticular formation, however their precise role is unknown.

Geniculate nuclei

The medial geniculate nucleus forms part of the auditory pathway and the lateral geniculate nucleus forms part of the visual pathway.

THE LIMBIC SYSTEM

The limbic system has traditionally been associated with our emotional behaviour, although areas outside the region are also implicated in this function, namely the amygdala and the medial and orbital aspects of the frontal lobe. Although some areas within the limbic system have various other functions, this section will concentrate only on the role of the limbic system in emotional behaviour.

Our emotional behaviour can be considered from two aspects, the control of a behaviour and the actual expression of that behaviour.

BASIC ANATOMY AND FUNCTION OF THE EXPRESSION OF EMOTIONAL BEHAVIOUR

Our emotional states are various but they all possess common attributes, namely visceral and somatic motor responses and powerful subjective feelings. Figure 9.2 shows a summary of this emotional motor response in terms of the level of control and the response intiated.

It is interesting that in different emotional states the pattern of the motor response from the autonomic system (involuntary movement) and voluntary movement is emotion specific. Recent studies indicate a strong link between the emotional state, the motor response (especially the facial expression) and the subjective experience.

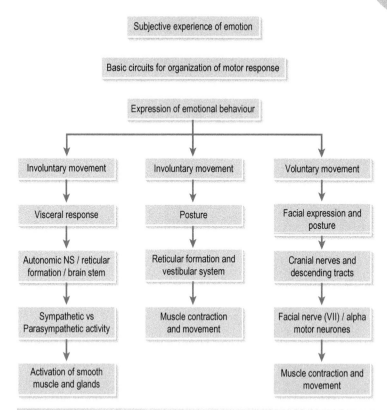

Figure 9.2 Summary of the emotional motor response.

Involuntary movement

Visceral motor response   This occurs as a result of changes in the autonomic nervous system (ANS), which is distributed throughout the central and peripheral nervous systems. The ANS can alter heart rate, respiratory rate, blood flow, piloerection, sweat gland activity and gastrointestinal motility. These responses occur via changes in smooth muscle, cardiac muscle and various glands throughout the body.

The ANS has two sub-divisions (sympathetic and parasympathetic) which produce the opposite affects on the body. This antagonistic action is essential in maintaining homeostasis (a stable internal environement) and is integrally linked with opposing emotional states.

Sympathetic nervous system   This initiates changes in the heart and lungs, smooth muscle of blood vessels, hair follicles, sweat

glands and abdominal organs in preparation for some kind of challenge/threat. The efferent output comes from the spinal cord, the paravertebral ganglia of the sympathetic trunk (Levels T_1 – $L_{2/3}$), to various ganglia/nuclei and onto effector glands/organs.
Parasympathetic nervous system (including the enteric division) This modifies the action of similar organs to the sympathetic division but its action is directed towards conserving and restoring energy. The efferent output comes from nuclei in the brain stem (cranial nerves III, VII, IX and X) and from the spinal cord grey matter (levels $S_{2/3/4}$) to various ganglia close to the organs that they innervate and onto the effector glands/organs.
Posture Alterations in posture associated with emotional behaviour occur in part via the vestibular system (S2.10) and the reticular formation (S2.10).

Voluntary movement
Movement related to facial expressions and postures associated with various emotions are clearly recognizable to most people and function as non-verbal communication about our emotional state.
Facial expression This is achieved by a highly coordinated output from the motor specific facial nerve (VII cranial nerve) (S2.10), which innervates all 20 of the muscles involved in facial expression (e.g. occiptal frontalis, orbicularis oris, buccinator, orbicularis oculi and platysma).
Posture and distal movement Voluntary changes in posture and fine control of distal movement also occur via voluntary control of the descending tracts (S2.14) to alpha motor neurons at all levels of the spinal cord.

BASIC ANATOMY AND FUNCTION OF THE CONTROL OF EMOTIONAL BEHAVIOUR
The control of our emotional behaviour is complex and involves many different structures. The two cerebral hemispheres make different contributions to the control of emotion. First, the right hemisphere is more important for the expression of emotion via the modulation of speech patterns, e.g. when we change the tone or volume of our voice to show anger. Damage to the region would leave the voice monotone and expressionless. Second, the left hemisphere has been found to be more involved with positive moods and the right with negative moods. This has implications in unilateral brain damage, which may result in inappropriate levels of depression (left-side damage) or elation (right-side damage).

The structures involved in control of our emotional behaviour are the:

Hypothalamus

Found in the temporal lobe, the hypothalamus is the centre for coordinating the voluntary and involuntary components of emotional behaviour. The main targets for the hypothalamus lie in the reticular formation which outputs to motor and autonomic effectors in the brain stem and spinal cord.

Cingulate gyrus

The cingulate gyrus lies in the frontal and parietal lobes and is involved in motor planning and regulation of cognitive and emotional processing via its link to the basal ganglia. The selection and initiation of behaviours is especially related to gaining reward and avoiding punishment.

Amygdala

The amygdala is found in the anteromedial temporal lobe and links the cortical regions that process sensory information with the effector systems of the hypothalamus and brain stem. Although it is not part of the limbic system, it has a major role in giving emotional significance to a sensory experience, especially visual stimuli. For example, an individual understanding that a nearby wild bear is associated with fear. Of course, the significance of a sensory experience is highly subjective and therefore specific to each individual. The amygdala can also influence the expression of emotion via both somatic and visceral systems.

Medial and orbital pre-frontal lobe

These regions are linked to the amygdala and integrate a combination of information from vision, somatosensory, olfactory and taste sensations.

Mamillary body

Found in the posterior temporal lobe, the mamillary body connects hypothalamus and cingulate cortex.

Although the following structures are considered to be part of the limbic system they have very little to do with emotional behaviour:

Hippocampus

Located in the medial temporal lobe, the hippocampus connects back to the hypothalamus via the fornix. This region is important in establishing new declarative memories.

Parahippocampus

The parahippocampus structure surrounds the hippocampus and has an important role in memory encoding and retrieval, especially of spatial memory (e.g. rooms and landscapes).

REFERENCES AND FURTHER READING

Klit H, Finnerup NB, Jensen TS: Central post-stroke pain: clinical characteristics pathophysiology and management, *The Lancet* 89:857–868, 2009.

Purves D, Augustine GJ, Fitzpatrick D, et al: *Neuroscience*, ed 4, Sunderland, 2008, Sinauer Associates.

Snell RS: *Clinical neuroanatomy*, ed 6, Philadelphia, 2006, Lippincott Williams and Wilkins.

Brain stem, cranial nerves, visual system, vestibular system, reticular system

BRAIN STEM

Although the brain stem incorporates many important structures, only the structures perceived to be most relevant to the therapist in terms of the neurologically impaired patient are discussed in this section.

BASIC ANATOMY

Anatomically, the brain stem is divided into three regions: the mid-brain, the pons and the medulla oblongata. Although the three regions have features which are common to all, they have others which allow us to distinguish between them.

Mid-brain

The mid-brain is approximately 1.5 cm long and extends from the pons to the mamillary bodies. The ventral surface connects to the two superior cerebellar peduncles (S2.12). The roof of the mid-brain is composed of four colliculi, the superior colliculi associated with the visual system and the inferior colliculi related to the auditory system. The red nucleus is also contained within the mid-brain. The periaqueductal grey, an area of grey matter within the mid-brain, is important in the descending modulation of pain (S3.29).

The following cranial nerves emerge from the mid-brain:

- Optic (II)
- Oculomotor (III)
- Trochlear (IV)

Pons

The pons is about 2.5 cm long and is composed of transverse fibres which form ridges across the surface of the area. The middle cerebellar peduncles attach to the pons.

The following cranial nerves emerge from the pons:

- Trigeminal (V)
- Abducens (VI)
- Facial (VII)
- Vestibulocochlear (VIII)

Medulla oblongata

The medulla is about 3 cm long and forms the base of the brain stem, adjoining the spinal cord at the level of foramen magnum. The descending motor tracts passing through it form two pyramids on the ventral surface of the medulla between which is the anterior median fissure. This fissure is disrupted where the tracts cross over the midline, termed the 'decussation of the pyramids'. The inferior cerebellar peduncle attaches to the medulla and behind it is the 'olive'. The olive is a prominent oval swelling that marks the position of the inferior olivary nucleus (S2.12).

The following cranial nerves emerge from the medulla:

- Glossopharyngeal (IX)
- Vagus (X)
- Accessory (XI)
- Hypoglossal (XII)

FUNCTION OF THE BRAIN STEM

The three regions of the brain stem contain the nuclei of the cranial nerves which control a variety of vital functions (S2.10). The ascending (S2.15) and descending tracts (S2.14) also pass through the brain stem between the spinal cord and cerebral cortex. The reticular formation (S2.10) and the cerebellum (S2.12) are integrally linked with all three regions and have specialist roles related to movement.

CRANIAL NERVES

BASIC ANATOMY

The names, numbers and functions of the cranial nerves can be seen in Table 10.1.

Motor nuclei

Five of the cranial nerves are entirely motor. Afferent input to the motor nuclei is from the cerebral cortex via the cortico-bulbar tract (S2.14). The output from the cranial nerve nuclei to the effector muscle is via a lower motor neuron.

Sensory nuclei

Three of the cranial nerves are entirely sensory. The afferent input is from the relevant sensory organ, e.g. the rods and cones of the retina for the optic nerve. They synapse in the brain stem in the relevant cranial nerve nuclei and finally decussate and ascend to other regions including the thalamus and ultimately the cerebral cortex.

Table 10.1 Names and functions of the cranial nerves

Cranial nerve	Motor/sensory/ mixed	Function of the cranial nerves
Olfactory (I)	S	Smell
Optic (II)	S	Vision – acuity and visual fields
Oculomotor (III)	Mo	Raises upper eyelid. Turns eyeball up, down and medially Parasympathetic output – iris constriction
Trochlear (IV)	Mo	Assists in turning eyeball down and laterally
Trigeminal (V)	Mix	
Ophthalmic division	S	Cornea, skin of forehead, scalp, eyelids and nose
Maxillary division	S	Skin over maxilla, teeth of upper jaw and palate
Mandibular division	Mo	Muscles of mastication and swallow. Tensor tympani (functions to reduce the amplitude of sounds)
	S	Skin of cheek, mandible and side of head. Teeth of lower jaw and temporomandibular joint. Anterior tongue
Abducens (VI)	Mo	Turns the eyeball laterally
Facial (VII)	Mix	
	Mo	Muscles of face and swallow
	S	Taste anterior $\frac{2}{3}$ of tongue
	Secretomotor	Parasympathetic control of salivary glands and lacrimal gland (tear duct)
Vestibulocochlear (VIII)	S	
Vestibular	S	From vestibular apparatus related to position and movement of head
Cochlear	S	Organ of hearing

Cranial nerve	Motor/sensory/ mixed	Function of the cranial nerves
Glossopharyngeal (IX)	Mix	
	Mo	Swallowing
	S	Taste posterior $\frac{1}{3}$ of tongue
	Secretomotor	Parasympathetic control of salivary gland
Vagus (X)	Mix	
	Mo	Parasympathetic innervation of heart and large blood vessels
	S	General sensation to lungs, larynx, trachea and bronchi, gastrointestinal tract, colon, liver and kidneys
Accessory (XI)	Mo	
Cranial root	Mo	Muscles of soft palate, some of the muscles of pharynx and larynx
Spinal root	Mo	Innervates sternocleidomastoid and trapezius
Hypoglossal (XII)	Mo	Muscles of tongue related to shape and movement

Mixed nuclei

The remaining four nuclei are mixed, sensory and motor, nerves.

Assessment of the cranial nerves

Traditionally, this has been carried out by the medical team on initial contact and is not covered in this text. However, it is important for the therapist to understand the findings and to identify any changes that may occur. Symptoms associated with cranial deficits may be identified by the patient themselves during the subjective assessment (S3.16) or noticed by the therapist by general observation (S3.17). In either case, any suspicions should be followed up with a referral to an experienced clinician or the medical team.

VISUAL SYSTEM

BASIC ANATOMY

The visual pathway

The sensory receptors of the visual system are the photosensitive rod and cone proteins of the retina. The rods and cones are most dense in the central region of the retina called the fovea. An image of the environment is focused onto the retina by alterations in the thickness of the lens. The retina converts a light pattern into a neuronal signal, which is conducted along the visual pathway to various parts of the brain to be processed (Fig. 10.1).

FUNCTION OF THE VISUAL SYSTEM

Binocular vision

This is defined as vision in which two eyes are used. Although there is a huge area of overlap between the visual fields of the left and right eye the eyes still view the environment slightly differently. The brain uses this slight disparity to estimate distance, allowing us to perceive 3D objects and spatial depth. If the two views are not successfully merged, the individual may develop double vision (diplopia).

Central or foveal vision

The fovea is responsible for sharp central vision necessary for any activity where visual detail is of primary importance. For example, reading and watching TV. Hence, if clarity is required, visual gaze must be centred on this region.

Peripheral vision

This aspect of vision occurs outside the centre of gaze and is weaker because the density of rods and cones outside the fovea region is much less. However, our peripheral vision is essential for fast reactions to visual stimuli in the periphery and monitoring body position relative to gravity. Our peripheral vision also allows the individual to recognize well-known structures and forms without the need to focus centrally.

Visual acuity

This is the clearness of vision and is achieved by the alteration of lens thickness and pupil size by small local muscles within the eyeball itself which focus the image at the fovea. However, acuity also relies upon coordination between head and body movements to ensure that the visual stimuli remains at fovea. This involves the ability to fix and scan.

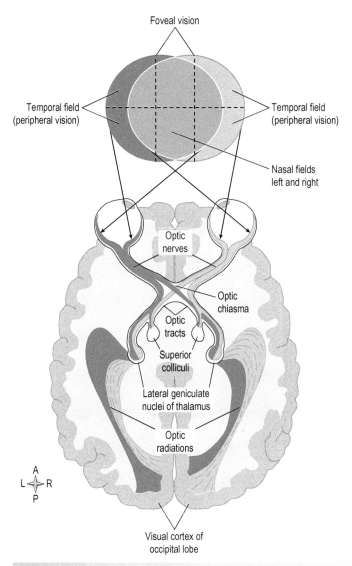

Figure 10.1 The visual pathway.

Fixing (S3.27)   The ability to fix gaze on an object while the body is moving, e.g. when travelling on a train or in a car. The mechanism can be explained as follows. When your head turns to the right, there is a slow reflex movement of your eyes to the left, in order that they appear to remain stationary. This is achieved via the vestibulocular reflex and as the name suggests, is under the direction of the vestibular system (S2.10). The effector muscles are innervated by the cranial nerve nuclei (III and VI).

Scanning (S3.27)   The ability to scan the eyes and head in a coordinated manner to maintain the object of interest or visual stimuli in the field of vision, e.g. while reading. The relevant head/neck movements are achieved via the tectospinal and tectobulbar tracts (S2.15) and eye movements by the cranial nerve nucleui (III and VI).

Visual fields (S3.27)

Information from the temporal and nasal visual fields of both eyes reaches the occipital cortex simultaneously, via the visual pathway (Fig. 10.1).

Visual perception

Vision provides the central nervous system with information related to our body position and the environment, however how we perceive and make sense of this raw information is highly subjective. The interpretation of our surroundings is integrally linked with memory and experience and therefore is individual in nature.

Vision and movement

The visual system plays an important part in movement and balance as it provides us with:

- A reference point to the vertical (visual proprioception) and spatial awareness
- The relationship between our body parts and our perception of midline during movement
- A comparison of our own self-motion and the movement of external objects.

However, we can of course balance without vision and vision can be unreliable. For example, our visual system is not always accurate when differentiating between self-motion and the movement of an external body. This may be observed when stationary in a car/bus/train and a vehicle pulls off alongside. Often, this can be perceived as self-motion and you may react accordingly, when actually it is the external object that is in motion.

VESTIBULAR SYSTEM

BASIC ANATOMY

The vestibular nuclei of the 8th cranial nerve are found within the pons and are the integrating centre for the vestibular system.

Input to the vestibular system

The sensory receptor of the vestibular system is the vestibular apparatus housed in the labyrinth of the inner ear – the labyrinth being made up of an outer bony labyrinth and an inner membraneous labyrinth full of endolymph. The labyrinth is divided into three sections, all of which function by translating movement of sensory hairs into electrical impulses:

Cochlear: which is associated with hearing and will not be discussed further here
Vestibule: known as the static labyrinth
Semicircular canals: known as the kinetic labyrinth.

Vestibule   The vestibule consists of two organs, the utricle and saccule. In the wall of the utricle and saccule is a thickened region of specialized epithelium, called a 'macula' (Fig. 10.2).

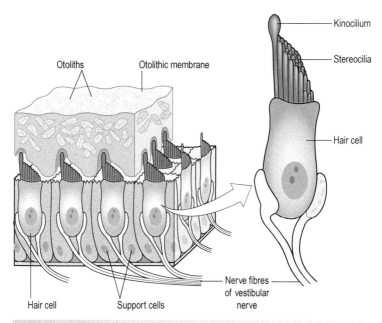

Figure 10.2 The structure of a macula.

The macula consists of two types of cells:

Supporting cells: Each supporting cell has a sensory neuron connection (vestibular branch of the vestibulocochlear nerve VIII). These cells secrete a thick gelatinous layer called the 'otolithic membrane' on top of which is a dense layer of calcium carbonate crystals called 'otoliths'. This characteristic is highly relevant to the receptors function.

Hair cell bundles (Fig. 10.2): Each supporting cell holds a bundle of hair cells, stereocilia (40–80/bundle) and kinocilium (1/bundle). Each stereocilia is physically connected to the kinocilium so that when it is moved, mechanically gated ion channels are opened allowing the movement of ions. This creates a graded potential in the sensory neuron. The cell is hyperpolarized when the stereocilia moves away from the kinocilium and depolarized with movement in the opposite direction.

The macula is divided into two halves with all of the hair bundles within one-half of the macula orientated in the same way. This ensures that a body movement, which leads to a graded potential in one hair bundle cell is likely to do the same in all the other cells and hence, guarantee an action potential in the sensory neuron. The hair bundles in the other half of the macula are all orientated in the opposite direction producing the opposite response and allowing the whole organ to be responsive to all relevant directions of movement. The macula orientation in the other side of the *brain* is the **same**, the relevance of this can be seen later in this section.

Semicircular canals   There are three semicircular canals which lie at 90° to each other. At the base of each canal is a thickened region termed the 'ampulla'. Inside the ampulla is an elevation of specialized cells called the 'crista' (Fig. 10.3).

The crista consists of two types of cells:

Supporting cells: The supporting cells are similar in structure to those of the macula. They produce a gel which overlies the hair bundles like a cap. This is termed the 'cupola' and it is much deeper than the otolithic membrane of the macula so that it covers the full width of the ampulla. This means that the endolymph within the membranous labyrinth cannot pass the cupola and it is this feature that is highly relevant to its function.

Hair cell bundles: The hair bundles are in the same arrangement as for the macula and are all orientated in the same direction within one canal. However, each canal has a

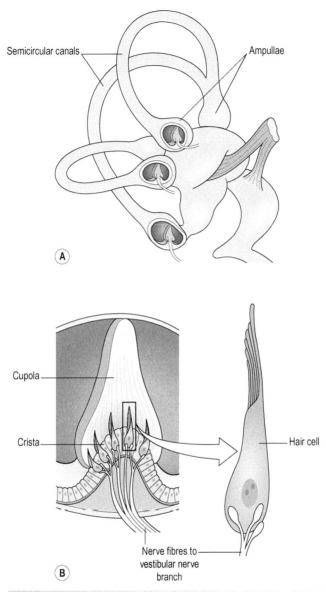

Figure 10.3 (A,B) The structure of a crista.

different orientation so that the semicircular canals can respond to movement in any plane. The orientation of the left and right sides of the *brain* is also **different** with each contralateral equivalent aligned in the opposite direction. The relevance of this will be explained below.

Output from the vestibular system

The vestibular system primarily works subcortically and has few synapses, therefore it responds very quickly, which is vital in terms of balance. From the vestibular apparatus, information passes along the vestibular nerve (VIII) and is processed at the vestibular nucleus in the pons. From here efferent connections go to the:

Cerebellum (S2.12) for processing and execution of smooth co-ordinated movement

Cranial nerves (III and VI) to initiate the vestibulo-ocular reflex

Descending tracts to initiate the appropriate muscle response. The muscle activation via the vestibulospinal tract will be specific to need but involving the neck, proximal limb and trunk muscles (lateral and medial vestibulospinal tract).

FUNCTION OF THE VESTIBULAR SYSTEM

Vestibule

The static labyrinth (utricle and saccule) detects linear movement by way of its sensory organ, the macula. The utricle detects linear movement in a frontal plane and the saccule in a sagittal plane.

The linear movement may be a result of *gravity*, e.g. head tilting or bending over to pick up an object from the floor or *linear translation* such as the acceleration and deceleration experienced when walking or travelling by car. In either case, the linear movement causes changes in the macula structure and consequently, a muscle action in terms of a balance response.

For example, during a forward head tilt (cervical spine flexion), the macula of the saccule will respond. The forward tilt causes the heavy mass of the otoliths and the otolithic membrane to 'fall' forwards moving the stereocilia in relation to the kinocilium and producing a graded potential in the sensory neuron. As the orientation of hair cells is opposite within each half of the saccule, the result will be depolarization (excitation) in one-half and hyperpolarization (inhibition) in the other (S2.6).

The action potential produced travels along the vestibular nerve (VIII) and recruits or inhibits the appropriate muscles via the vestibulospinal tract (S2.15). In this case, the forward head tilt has moved the centre of gravity forwards making the body less stable. The balance reaction required will attempt to bring the centre of gravity backwards, by recruiting extensor muscles around the pelvis/hip or trunk and simultaneously reduce the activity of the flexor muscles. This is important so that the centre of gravity is not moved further forwards and balance becomes seriously compromised. Remember also that the orientation of hair bundles in one-half of the saccule is the same in both the left and right sides of the brain and therefore the response will be bilateral. This makes sense, as the response to a linear movement needs to be symmetrical.

Semicircular canals

The kinetic labyrinth (semicircular canals) detects the movement of rotation in all planes, e.g. head rotation to look over your shoulder, or a somersault on a trampoline.

As with the static labyrinth, the movement occurring results in a muscle action response as a result of nerve cells being depolarized or hyperpolarized. However, the mechanism by which the sensory organ achieves this is slightly different.

As highlighted in the anatomy section, the cupola is the full width of the ampulla and this stops the free flow of endolymph within each canal. When a rotation movement is experienced, movement of the endolymph is blocked by the cupola producing a force upon the gel structure. The response of the hair bundles embedded in the cupola is as for the macula in terms of production of an action potential in the sensory nerve.

The hair bundles within one canal are all orientated the same way so that the response is sufficient to guarantee an action potential. In the semicircular canals, the orientation of one canal is different on the contralateral side of the brain and this is important because rotation is asymmetrical in nature and therefore requires a different motor response from each side of the body for balance to be maintained.

Assessment of the vestibular system

Rehabilitation of vestibular disorders is recognized as a specialist field in physiotherapy. Therefore, if a lesion of the vestibular system is suspected, referral to a specialist unit is advised. Assessment of the vestibular system is not covered in this text.

RETICULAR SYSTEM

BASIC ANATOMY

The reticular formation is a complicated network of circuits which extend from the spinal cord through the medulla, pons, mid-brain, subthalamus, hypothalamus and thalamus. Although previously considered anatomically ill-defined, more recent scientific investigation has shown the reticular formation to be well organized and functionally discrete. Anatomically it can be conveniently divided into three longitudinal columns:

- The median column consisting of intermediate sized neurons
- The medial column containing large neurons (the median and medial columns are also known as the raphe nuclei)
- The lateral column mainly consisting of smaller neurons.

Afferent connections

Afferent information enters the reticular formation from most parts of the central nervous system. Most notably:

- Spinal cord (S2.13)
- Cranial nerves (S2.10)
- Cerebellum (S2.12)
- Limbic system (S2.9)
- Cerebral cortex (motor and sensory areas) (S2.7).

Efferent connections

The reticular formation projects to all levels of the central nervous system including most of the cerebral cortex. Most notably:

- Cerebellum (S2.12)
- Cranial nerves (S2.10)
- Motor pathways of the spinal cord (S2.13, 14).

FUNCTION OF THE RETICULAR FORMATION

Cardiovascular and respiratory control

The cardiorespiratory centres are now considered part of the reticular formation. In terms of respiratory function, many of the neurons from the reticular formation synapse on motor neurons that innervate the muscles of inspiration and expiration. The control of cardiovascular function is via regulation of the autonomic system (a) parasympathetic output from the vagus nerve and (b) sympathetic output from the sympathetic trunk levels T_{1-5} of the spinal cord.

Modulation of muscle tone

The appropriate level of resting muscle tone is regulated by modulation of the stretch reflex (S2.13) by the descending tracts. The reticulospinal tracts in combination with the vestibulospinal and reticulobulbar tracts influence muscle tone at the level of the alpha motor neuron. The two reticulospinal tracts specifically influence extensor muscle tone. The pontine/lateral reticulospinal tract terminates at the ventral horn directly on motor neurons and enhances extensor muscle tone, whereas the medullary/medial reticulospinal tract (S2.14) terminates indirectly on motor neurons and exerts an inhibitory influence on extensor muscle tone. The antagonistic effect of these tracts allows modulation and grading to set the level of extensor muscle tone appropriately for the functional need. However, the reticulospinal tracts also work in cooperation with the vestibulospinal tracts (S2.14) to specifically maintain tone of the antigravity muscles.

The reticular formation also has a role in the motor control of facial expression related to our emotional behaviour (S2.9) via its links to the limbic system and coordination of the timing and direction of eye movements via the superior colliculus and cranial nerves.

Pain modulation

The reticular formation has a key role in modulating pain perception (S3.29).

Regulation of the sleep/wake cycle

Our normal sleep/wake cycle shows a definite recognizable daily pattern, with the hypothalamus being ultimately involved in its control. However connections to the hypothalamus allow the reticular formation to influence these biological rhythms. The role of the reticular formation in this function is not wholly understood, however the reticular activating system (RAS), which lies near the junction of the pons and mid-brain, appears to be the primary cause of wakefulness and rapid eye movement (REM) sleep. REM sleep is characterized by an increase in brain activity and an inactive body. On the other hand, inactivity of the RAS region, via inhibition from the hypothalamus is important for producing non-REM sleep, a stage of deep sleep characterized by an active body and reduced brain activity.

REFERENCES AND FURTHER READING

Hunziker H-W: *In the eye of the reader: foveal and peripheral perception – from letter recognition to the joy of reading,* Zürich, 2006, Transmedia Stäubli Verlag.

Palmer SM, Rosa MG: A distinct anatomical network of cortical areas for analysis of motion in far peripheral vision, *European Journal of Neuroscience* 248:2389–2405, 2006.

Purves D, Augustine GJ, Fitzpatrick D, et al: *Neuroscience,* ed 4, Sunderland, 2008, Sinauer Associates.

Snell RS: *Clinical neuroanatomy,* ed 6, Philadelphia, 2006, Lippincott Williams and Wilkins.

Basal ganglia

BASIC ANATOMY

FUNCTION OF THE BASAL GANGLIA
Function of the BG in motor control

The big picture
The detail
Function in motor learning

BASIC ANATOMY

The functional nuclei of the basal ganglia (BG) include:

- Striatum (caudate nucleus and putamen), which receives information from all parts of the cerebral cortex except the primary visual and auditory cortices
- Globus pallidus internus (GPi)
- Globus pallidus externus (GPe)
- Subthalamic nucleus (STN)
- Substantia nigra (SN) – pars reticulata (pr) and pars compacta (pc) which contain dopamine-producing cells.

The circuitry between these functional nuclei forms several pathways, the direct, indirect and hyperdirect, the arrangement of which can be seen in Figure 11.1. The BG is also *topographically arranged* with each body part represented relative to its innervations.

FUNCTION OF THE BASAL GANGLIA

In basic terms, the BG functions as a selection processor by filtering the vast amount of input it receives and selecting an appropriate response in relation to both novel and well learned movement sequences. By the same process it is also instructive in terms of the *planning*, *initiation* and *execution* of these movements. This filtering occurs through the interaction of the three pathways described above on the output nucleus, the GPi. It is estimated that 1 million cortical cells synapse upon each GPi cell.

As well as the motor loop shown in Figure 11.1, there are three other loops within the BG which have their origins in different cortical areas and carry out specific functions via similar circuitry. Although previously described as discrete parallel loops, recent evidence indicates that there is a high level of interaction between these loops. However, the selection function described above is true for all of them, the motor loop (voluntary movement or learning), the limbic loop (emotions) and the associative loop (cognition and sensory integration). Based on its anatomical connections with the nociceptive system, the BG is also considered crucial in pain modulation. It appears that the interaction of several of these loops make it possible for the BG to influence several dimensions of pain (sensory discrimination, affective and

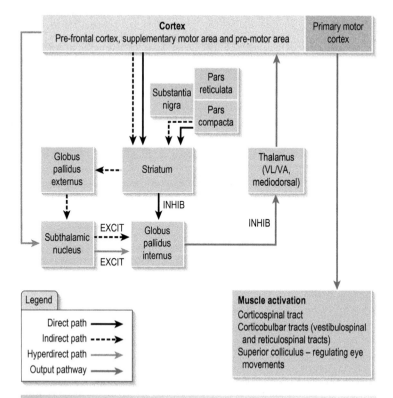

Figure 11.1 The basic anatomical arrangement of the basal ganglia.

cognitive) as well as the modulation of pain itself via its filtering role.

FUNCTION OF THE BG IN MOTOR CONTROL

The big picture

The pre-frontal cortex (S2.7) provides an idea for movement, a goal, based upon the internal and external environment. A relevant movement plan is selected from learned stored programmes in the supplementary motor area (SMA) and pre-motor area (PMA) (S2.7). At this stage, the BG assists in the selection of an appropriate plan, its initiation and termination. The selected plan is returned to the SMA and PMA for future reference and to the primary motor cortex from which the plan is executed via the descending tracts (S2.14).

The detail

The anatomical connections of the three pathways within the BG can be seen in Figure 11.1. Before exploring the detailed workings of how the BG achieves its function, a brief description of the role of each pathway is necessary. In essence, the *direct pathway* allows the selected motor programme through to the thalamus and is responsible for initiating the plan, while the *indirect pathway* halts any unwanted motor programmes and terminates the plan. These two pathways are also modulated by the SNpc circuit at the level of the striatum (Fig. 11.1). The neurotransmitter dopamine released by the SNpc cells has the opposite effect on the neurons of each pathway. It is excitatory to the direct pathway, reinforcing its action and is inhibitory to the indirect pathway so reducing its action. In both cases, this results in more chance of a motor programme being released to the thalamus when the SNpc neurons are active. Recent evidence has indicated the existence of a third pathway termed the *hyperdirect* (Fig. 11.1) which links the cortex directly to the STN and on to the GPi. This pathway is considered to be faster conducting than either the direct or indirect pathways. Its role is the same as the indirect pathway. Ultimately, it is the balance of activity between these three pathways at the GPi that acts as the filtering system to ensure the appropriate selection of a movement programme. The relative contribution of each of these pathways is at present unknown.

The intricate circuitry of the BG is highly complex but the following highlights the basics in a normal nervous system.

At rest   There is no input from the cortex but as the GPi is spontaneously active it therefore switches off (inhibits) any thalamic activity. The result is no movement.

During movement There is stimulation from the cortex. The cortex is sending motor programmes to the BG for correct selection and implementation. This occurs as follows:

Selection of the appropriate motor programme. The decision as to the appropriate motor programme to select is based upon internal cues from the huge amount of sensory input received by the BG. Whether the programme is selected or not has recently been attributed to the competition/balance between the direct and indirect/hyperdirect pathways:

- In the *direct pathway*, the striatum *stops* the GPi from *switching off* the thalamus (to stop inhibition is termed 'disinhibition') and results in the release of the selected motor programme by the thalamus
- In the *hyperdirect* (via the cortex) and *indirect* (via the striatum) *pathways*, the GPi is excited or *switched on* so that again it *stops* the thalamus releasing any information and this results in unwanted motor programmes being halted.

Initiation and termination of the selected programme. This is achieved by adjusting the specific timing of activation of the three pathways:

- The hyperdirect pathway, which is fast conducting, excites or *switches on* the GPi so stopping the programme from being released by the thalamus
- Next, the direct pathway stops the GPi inhibiting the thalamus so allowing the selected programme to be initiated
- Finally, the indirect pathway switches on the GPi, to stop any further information leaving the thalamus and thus terminates the motor programme.

FUNCTION IN MOTOR LEARNING

Recent evidence suggests that the BG is also involved in motor learning. The dopaminergic neurons of the SNpc are thought to have the ability to induce neuroplastic changes in the neurons between the cortex and the striatum. These changes are facilitated in line with reward/reinforcement of a successful voluntary movement with synaptic efficacy being increased within the relevant pathways (direct, indirect and hyperdirect). Therefore, during future use the successful programme will be selected more automatically.

REFERENCES AND FURTHER READING

Boecker H, Jankowski J, Ditter P, et al: A role of the basal ganglia and midbrain nuclei for initiation of motor sequences, *Neuroimage* 39:1356–1369, 2008.

Cunnington R, Windischberger C, Deecke L, et al: The preparation and execution of self-initiated and externally-triggered movement: a study of event related fMRI, *Neuroimage* 15:373–385, 2002.

Cunnington R, Windischberger C, Moser E: Premovement activity of the presupplementary motor area and the readiness for action: studies of time-resolved event-related functional MRI, *Human Movement Science* 24:644–656, 2005.

Elsinger CL, Harrington DL, Rao SM: From preparation to online control: reappraisal of neural circuitry mediating internally generated and externally guided actions, *Neuroimage* 31:1177–1187, 2006.

Graybiel AM: The basal ganglia: learning new tricks and loving it, *Current Opinion in Neurobiology* 15:638–644, 2005.

Gerardin E, Pochon JB, Poline JB, et al: Distinct striatal regions support movement selection preparation and execution, *Neuroreport* 15:2327–2331, 2004.

Haber SN, Calzavara R: The cortico-basal ganglia integrative network: the role of the thalamus, *Brain Research Bulletin* 78:69–74, 2009.

Jankowski J, Scheef L, Hüppe C, et al: Distinct striatal regions for planning and executing novel and automated movement sequences, *Neuroimage* 44:1369–1379, 2009.

Leblois A, Boraud T, Meissner W, et al: Competition between feedback loops underlies normal and pathological demands in the basal ganglia, *Journal of Neuroscience* 2613:3567–3583, 2008.

Nambu A: A new dynamic model of the cortico-basal ganglia loop, *Progress in Brain Research* 143:461–466, 2004.

Nambu A: Seven problems on the basal ganglia, *Current Opinion in Neurobiology* 18:595–604, 2008.

Nambu A, Tokuno H, Takada M: Functional significance of the cortico-subthalamo-pallidal 'hyperdirect' pathway, *Neuroscience Research* 43:111–117, 2008.

Melrose RJ, Poulin RM, Stern CE: An fMRI investigation of the role of the basal ganglia in reasoning, *Brain Research* 1142:146–158, 2007.

Monchi O, Petrides M, Strafella AP, et al: Functional role of the basal ganglia in the planning and execution of actions, *Annals of Neurology* 59:257–264, 2006.

Pasupathy A, Miller EK: Different time courses of learning-related activity in the prefrontal cortex and striatum, *Nature* 433:873–876, 2005.

Smith Y, Raju D, Nanda B, et al: The thalamostriatal systems: anatomical and functional organization in normal and parkinsonian states, *Brain Research Bulletin* 78:60–68, 2009.

The Parkinson's Disease Society: *The professional's guide to Parkinson's disease*, 2007. www.parkinsons.org.uk/PDF/PubProfessionalGuideNov07pdf.

Weilke F, Spiegel S, Boecker H, et al: Time-resolved fMRI of activation patterns in M1 and SMA during complex voluntary movement, *Journal of Neurophysiology* 85:1858–1863, 2001.

Cerebellum

BASIC ANATOMY

The cerebellum, often refered to as the 'little brain', makes up only 10% of the total brain volume but contains more than 50% of the total number of neurons. It is composed of an outer layered cortical region and an inner subcortical mass of cells which form the deep cerebellar nuclei (DCN). The cerebellum is topographically arranged and has *ipsilateral* control of movement, that is, the left hemisphere of the cerebellum controls the left side of the body. The cerebellum is divided by two deep transverse fissures into three lobes, anterior, posterior and flocculonodular lobe. On the upper surface there are three functional regions separated anatomically by two longtitudinal stripes. The central vermis (medial zone) and two paravermal regions or hemispheres. The paravermal regions are divided into the lateral and intermediate zones.

THE DEEP CEREBELLAR NUCLEI
There are four deep cerebellar nuclei (DCN):

- Fastigial
- Interposed – globose and emboliform
- Dentate

All output from the cerebellum leaves via the DCN, with the exception of output to the vestibular nuclei which has a direct connection. Afferent pathways also send collaterals that synapse on neurons in the DCN.

THE FUNCTIONAL LOOPS

Based on its function, the cerebellum can be broadly divided into four loops:

The cerebrocerebellum

This incorporates a loop between the cerebral cortex and the cerebellum. It is located in the lateral zone of the paravermal regions and is strongly connected with the dentate nucleus.

The vestibulocerebellum

This incorporates a loop between the vestibular system and the cerebellum. It roughly corresponds to the flocculonodular lobe and has no connection to the DCN.

The spinocerebellum

This incorporates a loop between the spinal cord and the cerebellum. It extends through the central vermis (medial zone) linked to the fastigial nucleus and the intermediate zone of the paravermal regions connected to the interposed nucleus.

The olivocerebellum

This incorporates a loop between the inferior olivary nucleus (in the medulla oblongata) and the cerebellum. It has strong links to the DCN.

PEDUNCLES

The cerebellum is connected to the rest of the central nervous system by three bundles of nerves or pathways termed 'peduncles'. The superior peduncle carries almost entirely efferent information away from the cerebellum. The middle peduncles, of which there are two, carry afferent information into the cerebellum. The inferior peduncle carries both afferent and efferent information.

AFFERENT CONNECTIONS

The cerebellum receives information from many sources. Figure 12.1 shows the main afferent connections. Note that the vestibular and spinal inputs to the cerebellum remain ipsilateral as the information conveyed from these sources is also ipsilateral. However, the inputs from the cerebral cortex and the inferior

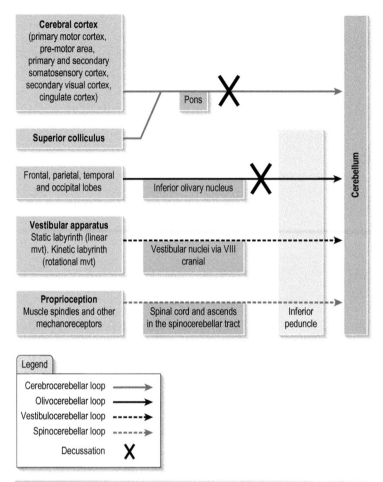

Figure 12.1 The afferent connections of the cerebellum.

olive (which contralateral) need to decussate (cross-over) before entering the cerebellum.

EFFERENT CONNECTIONS

The efferent connections from the cerebellum are shown in Figure 12.2. Note that the pathway to the vestibular nuclei is a direct projection, however all other efferent pathways exit the cerebellum by one of the DCN.

The axons from the dentate nucleus must again decussate to ensure the cerebral cortex receives information related to the

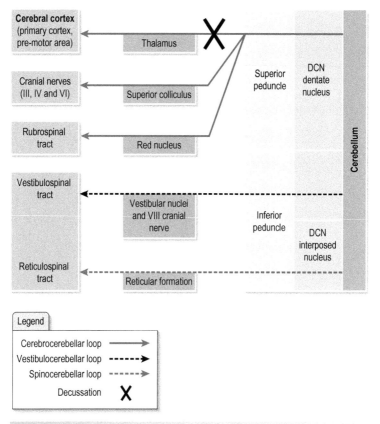

Figure 12.2 The efferent connections of the cerebellum.

appropriate side of the body. Output is ultimately destined to influence the the descending tracts which will innervate the relevant muscles for movement.

THE INTRINSIC CIRCUITRY WITHIN THE CEREBELLUM

Somatosensory information remains topographically arranged within the cerebellum although less organized than that of the cerebral cortex. Histologically, the cerebellum is organized into five cell layers which form a modulatory circuit throughout the cerebellar cortex. This circuitry is highly complex and beyond the scope of this book. However, in brief, the cells involved are:

Mossy fibres, which transmit information into the cerebellum.

Granule cells, which form parallel fibres and make thousands of contacts with a Purkinje cell. This system also has a collateral which is excitatory to the DCN.

Purkinje cells, which transmit information out of the cerebellum. These cells are inhibitory at the DCN.

Climbing fibres, which form the inferior olivary nucleus. One climbing fibre has many excitatory contacts with one Purkinje cell and is excitatory to the DCN.

Basket cells, stellate cells, Golgi cells, which are found only **within** the cerebellar cortex and are inhibitory in output.

In brief, the cerebellar circuitry forms a loop between the input neurons (mossy fibres and granule cells/parallel fibres and climbing fibres) and the output neurons (Purkinje cells) (Fig. 12.3) – the final output being via the DCN. The Golgi, stellate and basket cells work as *interneurons* to control/modulate the flow of information through this loop with their inhibitory contacts on the Purkinje cell. Also, the whole circuit has various other connections which allow it to be self-modulating. The final output is decided by the balance of excitation and inhibition at the DCN (granule cell and climbing fibres excitatory and Purkinje cell inhibitory).

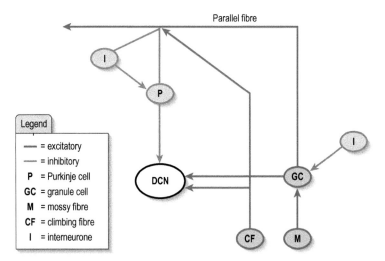

Figure 12.3 Summary of the intrinsic circuitry of the cerebellum.

FUNCTION OF THE CEREBELLUM

The three regions of the cerebellum have similar intrinsic circuitry (Fig. 12.3) but different functions which are a consequence of the origins and destinations of the input and output neurons, respectively. In brief, the cerebrocerebellum loop provides the cerebellum with knowledge about the intended plan for movement and the vestibulocerebellum and spinocerebellum loops monitor the actual position and motion of the body during the movement. Any mismatch/error is corrected and the movement is refined in terms of both timing and magnitude to meet the original goal. The correction is managed directly or indirectly via various descending tracts.

CEREBROCEREBELLUM

This loop is specifically involved in the regulating, planning and timing of movement. Its connections with the superior colliculus also give it a role in visually guided coordination of voluntary movement. In addition, it has a further role in regulating distal limb movment and speech, with damage to the region presenting as limb ataxia (S3.18, 26) and dysarthria (S3.16), respectively.

VESTIBULOCEREBELLUM

This loop is important in the regulation of posture and balance (S3.18, 32) via axial muscle control and vestibular reflexes. It also governs the eye movements associated with equilibrium (vestibulo-ocular reflex) (S2.10).

SPINOCEREBELLUM

This loop is primarily involved in the execution and control of axial and proximal muscle activity via the medial descending tracts. Therefore a role in postural control and balance is likely. Not surprisingly, damage to the area results in trunk ataxia (S3.26) but damage to the more lateral areas of the intermediate zone may also present with limb ataxia. The spinocerebellum also influences the level of muscle tone via the reticular system (S3.21). Recent studies are also challenging the view that this region participates only in the execution of movement and suggests that the intermediate zone also has a role in predictive control and adaptation.

The detail

The error correction system of the cerebellum is a consequence of modulation by the intrinsic circuitry. This forms the basis for regulation of movement as it occurs and over the longer term to initiate the changes that underly motor learning. This regulation occurs by altering the firing frequency of the Purkinje cells to ultimately influence the excitatory output at the DCN. The Purkinje cells and DCN are both tonically active at rest. During movement, there is a change in the rate of firing of these cells, the pattern of which exactly represents the movement being performed. The patterns of firing that are concurrently available to both cells are compared. Any error is corrected by altering the firing pattern, the Purkinje cells modulating (through inhibitory contacts) the excitatory output of DCN. A correct signal is then sent to the appropriate motor neurons to improve the accuracy of the movement. This provides an ongoing corrective mechanism while movement is occuring. Over time, the climbing fibres change the firing patterns via long-term depression (neuroplasticity) to reflect the corrected pattern of movement. In simple terms, the error has been corrected immediately during the movement and over time removed from the circuit; learning has occurred.

REFERENCES AND FURTHER READING

Ausim AS: And the olive said to the cerebellum: organization and functional significance of the olivo-cerebellar system, *The Neuroscientist* 13:616–626, 2007.

Bakker M, Allum JH, Visser JE, et al: Postural responses to multidirectional stance perturbations in cerebellar ataxia, *Experimental Neurology* 202:21–35, 2006.

Bastian AJ: Learning to predict the future: the cerebellum adapts feedforward movement control, *Current Opinion in Neurobiology* 16:645–649, 2006.

Ilg W, Giese MA, Gizewski ER, et al: The influence of focal cerebellar lesions on the control and adaptation of gait, *Brain* 131:2913–2927, 2008.

Kandel ER, Schwartz JH, Jessell TM: *Principles of neural science*, ed 4, New York, 2000, McGraw-Hill Health Professions Division.

Lo YL, Fook-Chong S, Chan LL, et al: Cerebellar control of motor activation and cancellation in humans: an electrophysiological study, *The Cerebellum* 8:302–311, 2009.

Ohki M, Kitazawa H, Hiramatsu T, et al: The role of primate cerebellar hemisphere in voluntary eye movement control revealed by lesion effects, *Journal of Neurophysiology* 101:934–947, 2009.

Purves D, Augustine GJ, Fitzpatrick D, et al: *Neuroscience*, Sunderland, 2008, Sinauer Associates.

Schoch B, Dimitrova A, Gizewski AB, et al: Functional localization in the human cerebellum based on voxelwise statistical analysis: a study of 90 patients, *Neuroimage* 30:36–51, 2006.

Shadmehr R, Krakauer JW: A computational neuroanatomy for motor control, *Experimental Brain Research* 185:359–381, 2008.

Timmann D, Konczak J, Ilg W, et al: Current advances in lesion-symptom mapping of the human cerebellum, *Neuroscience* 1:1–16, 2009.

Voogd J, Barmack NH: Oculomotor cerebellum, *Progress in Brain Research* 151:231–268, 2005.

13 The spinal cord and spinal reflexes

BASIC ANATOMY AND FUNCTION OF THE SPINAL CORD

GROSS ANATOMY

The spinal cord begins superiorly at the foramen magnum where it is continuous with the medulla oblongata (S2.10). It continues inferiorly within the vertebral column protected in the vertebral canal by the meninges and cerebrospinal fluid (S2.8). The lowest part of the spinal cord lies at the first lumbar vertebra (level $L_{1/2}$). Along the length of the spinal cord, there are two swollen regions: the cervical and lumbar enlargements, which represent the origins of the brachial and lumbosacral plexus, respectively.

GREY AND WHITE MATTER

In cross-section (Fig. 13.1), the spinal cord can be seen to consist of the inner grey matter (H shaped) and the remaining area

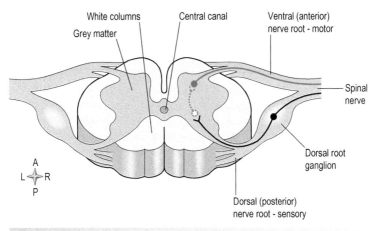

Figure 13.1 A cross-section of the spinal cord.

termed the white matter. These are so named because of their microscopic appearance and a consequence of the cells located within the area. The white matter consists of myelinated axons and represents the existence of the ascending and descending tracts (S2.14, 15). The grey matter is formed by the cell bodies of the same neurons and includes motor neurons and many interneurons which make connections within segments and between segments of the spinal cord. The grey matter is described in terms of the anterior/ventral horn and posterior/dorsal horn (Fig. 13.1). In the thoracic and upper lumbar region there is also a lateral horn, which represents the sympathetic trunk, part of the autonomic nervous system.

CENTRAL PATTERN GENERATORS (CPG)

A central pattern generator is a network of neurons within the spinal cord which underlie the production of most of our rhythmic motor output, such as walking, chewing/swallowing and breathing. These are by nature stereotyped, repetitive and complex movements but unlike reflex activity, are still under voluntary control. The network of neurons is thought to work in two opposing halves which when activated switch each other on and off to create a repetitive rhythmic action. The stereotyped movement pattern created avoids the need for descending commands from higher centres, however changes in the environment may require the CPG to be modulated and adapted to meet the changing needs. This modulation primarily comes from the higher centres but the CPGs also modulate themselves by responding to sensory feedback from the body. A small change in function may result in a long-term change to the whole CPG network as it adapts to achieve a motor goal. In terms of neurologically impaired patients, this may be positive or negative in relation to function.

SPINAL NERVES

At each spinal level there are a pair (left and right) of spinal nerves which exit the vertebral canal via the intervertebral foramen. There are 31 pairs of spinal nerves in total (8 cervical, 12 thoracic, 5 lumbar and 5 sacral). The spinal nerve consists of a sensory root and motor root (Fig. 13.1) from the spinal cord. The sensory root transmits information into the spinal cord and its cell body is found in the dorsal root ganglion just adjacent to the spinal cord but within the vertebral canal. The motor root carries information out of the spinal cord and its cell body is located in the anterior/ventral horn of the grey matter of the spinal cord. The sensory and motor roots at one level combine to form a spinal nerve and are part of the peripheral nervous system. Spinal nerves from several levels of the spinal cord will combine to form a peripheral nerve. For example, the median nerve consists of the spinal nerves from levels $C_{5/6/7/8}$ and T_1, whereas the musculocutaneous nerve includes spinal nerves from levels $C_{5/6/7}$.

CAUDA EQUINUS

From lumbar level $L_{1/2}$, where the spinal cord terminates the anatomy, is different. The cord itself is referred to as the 'cauda equinus' and represents a bundle of spinal roots from the segments above within the vertebral canal. This occurs because the vertebral column grows longer than the spinal cord during development. Therefore in the adult, the spinal cord segments do not correspond to the vertebral segment of the same level. For example, the lower lumbar and sacral spinal nerves exit at the appropriate levels (i.e. $L_{3/4/5}$ and S_{1-5}), however their spinal cord segments are found between T_9 and L_2 vertebral segments. This is important when considering pathologies which affect the spinal cord.

LOWER MOTOR NEURON/FINAL COMMON PATHWAY AND UPPER MOTOR NEURON

Understanding the anatomy of the spinal cord and its divisions is vital for ensuring your assessment of a neurologically impaired patient is appropriate and accurate. One important division is the differentiation between an upper motor neuron and lower motor neuron pathology and their clinical presentations.

The lower motor neuron/final common pathway

The neurons indicated as nerve roots in Figure 13.1 are the starting point of the lower motor neuron division. Anything more peripheral is included in this division. In effect, damage to these neurons is interpreted as a deficit of the peripheral nervous system, for example, Guillain–Barré syndrome and motor neuron disease. However, different clinical presentations can occur within this division depending upon the location of the lesion. For example, damage to the spinal root or spinal nerve would present very differently to that of a peripheral nerve.

Spinal root or spinal nerve   A single spinal root or nerve could be damaged with a very specific injury such as an intervertebral disc prolapse or in association with other trauma. The injury itself could relate to:

The sensory root carrying sensory information from a specific area of skin, termed a 'dermatome' (S3.24) *or*
The motor root innervating part of a muscle, termed a 'myotome' (S3.31) *or*
Both sensory and motor roots.

Therefore the clinical presentation resulting from damage to a single spinal root or spinal nerve will be very localized in terms of reduced sensation and/or a weakness in a specific muscle. Total paralysis of a muscle is unlikely as a single spinal root level innervates only a fraction of the muscle. For example, the triceps brachii muscle is supplied by the radial nerve ($C_{5/6/7/8}$ and T_1), so damage to root level C_5 would present as mild weakness and not total paralysis because the muscle is still innervated by the remaining undamaged spinal root levels.

Peripheral nerve   As already stated, the peripheral nerve consists of both sensory and motor spinal nerves from various spinal levels and in different combinations. Therefore a complete severance of a peripheral nerve will present with more widespread sensory and motor loss and even the complete paralysis of a muscle. The clinical presentation will be more diffuse, dictated by the individual peripheral nerve involved and whether the severance is complete or partial. For example, a complete lesion of the musculocutaneous nerve ($C_{5/6/7}$) in the upper arm would lead to complete paralysis of coracobrachialis, biceps brachii and brachialis muscles and loss of sensation in the area of skin supplied by its cutaneous branch.

The upper motor neuron

The upper motor neuron division includes any neuron that is confined entirely to the central nervous system. It includes any neuron between the brain and the peripheral nervous system, incorporating neurons within the spinal cord, the ascending and descending tracts and higher centres, such as the brain stem and cerebral cortex. Damage to the upper motor neuron pathway occurs in pathologies such as spinal cord injury, cerebrovascular accident, multiple sclerosis and Parkinson's disease. The central nervous system is highly complex and therefore, damage within this division could result in a wide range of diverse symptoms.

BASIC ANATOMY AND FUNCTION OF SPINAL REFLEXES

A reflex is an involuntary, almost instantaneous movement, in response to a stimulus that does not require the higher centres of the brain. However, information received from both the periphery and higher centres is used to modulate the reflex activity at the level of the spinal cord.

The neural pathway involved in a simple reflex arc includes:

Sensory receptor: This detects a stimulus
Afferent neuron: This transmits information from the periphery to the spinal cord
Integrating centre: This modulates the response of the reflex
Efferent neuron: This transmits information from the spinal cord to the periphery (effector organ)
Effector organ: This carries out the reflex response and is usually a muscle or a gland.

The most important reflex arcs in relation to movement control are:

● Stretch reflex
● Golgi tendon organ
● Flexor withdrawal and crossed extensor reflex.

STRETCH REFLEX

The stretch reflex has both a phasic and a tonic component. The phasic component adapts rapidly to a stimulus and responds to a *change* in muscle length. The tonic component which is continually active is more responsive to a constant stretch.

Phasic stretch reflex

This component of the stretch reflex is primarily monosynaptic:

Sensory receptor: A muscle spindle (dynamic nuclear bag), which responds to changes in length (stretch)

Afferent neuron: Type Ia afferent neurons enter the spinal cord through the dorsal horn and synapse in the grey matter directly on the efferent neuron

Efferent neuron: Alpha motor neuron (AMN)

Effector: Contraction of the same muscle from which the stretch was detected and any relevant synergist muscles required.

Function The phasic component is evident in the intact nervous system at rest and is the component that is assessed during reflex testing (S3.22). An imposed stretch on the muscle by the clinician gives information on nerve integrity and the reflexic properties of muscle. This technique is referred to as a tendon jerk.

Tonic stretch reflex (TSR)

This component is primarily polysynaptic:

Sensory receptor: A muscle spindle (nuclear chain or static nuclear bag), which responds to changes in length (stretch)

Afferent neuron: Type II afferent neurons enter the spinal cord through the dorsal horn and synapse in the grey matter on interneurons

Integrating centre: Excitatory interneurons within the grey matter of the spinal cord which synapse upon the AMN

Efferent neuron: Alpha motor neuron

Effector: Contraction of the same muscle from which the stretch was detected and any relevant synergist muscles required.

Function The tonic component is not apparent in an intact nervous system unless the muscle is already contracting. The TSR serves to set resting muscle tone (S3.21), the base level of muscle activity. The reflex arc also responds to changes in the environment adjusting the level of activity as appropriate to functional needs, e.g. lowering muscle activity when we lie down and raising it in preparation to stand up against gravity.

GOLGI TENDON ORGAN (GTO)

This reflex arc is polysynaptic:

Sensory receptor: Golgi tendon organ, which responds to changes in tension at the musculotendinous junction

Afferent neuron: Type Ib afferent neurons enter the spinal cord through the dorsal horn and synapse in the grey matter on an interneuron

Integrating centre: Inhibitory interneurons within the grey matter of the spinal cord

Efferent neuron: Alpha motor neuron

Effector: Reduced contraction of the same muscle from which the tension was detected.

Function This reflex is protective in terms of reducing a muscle contraction in circumstances where excessive tension is being produced and injury is likely. The GTO works in opposition to the TSR arc. Therefore, the balance of the two outputs at the alpha motor neuron ensures the level of muscle activity/tone is appropriate at rest and during movement without the risk of excessive tension and potential damage occurring. The GTO and TSR also provide the central nervous system with continuous information about the mechanical state of the muscle.

FLEXOR WITHDRAWAL AND CROSSED EXTENSOR REFLEX

This reflex is polysynaptic and initiated from the flexor withdrawal arc:

Sensory receptor: Free nerve endings (pain) in the plantar aspect of the foot

Afferent neuron: Type A delta afferent neurons enter the spinal cord through the dorsal horn and synapse in the grey matter on an interneuron

Integrating centre: Excitatory interneuron

Efferent neuron: Alpha motor neuron

Effector: Contraction of the flexor muscles of the ipsilateral lower limb.

Function The primary function of the flexor withdrawal reflex is protection in response to a painful stimulus. The crossed extensor reflex is supportive to this role as it simultaneously activates the extensor muscles of the contralateral lower limb for weight bearing, so that the ipsilateral lower limb can be flexed without the body falling over. There is some evidence to support the theory that this reflex also underlies our walking pattern, with alternating phases of stance (crossed extensor) and swing (flexor withdrawal).

ADDITIONAL NEURONAL ACTIVITY ASSOCIATED WITH THE REFLEX ARC

For the reflex arcs described above, additional circuitry exists to ensure the efficiency of the response and allow modification as necessary.

First, the afferent neuron within the circuit includes the following branches which synapse upon:

- An inhibitory interneuron within the spinal cord, which inhibits the AMN of the antagonist muscle so that the effector muscle is not contested. This is termed *reciprocal innervation*.
- A second order neuron of the ascending tract (dorsal columns) (S2.15), which transmits information to the higher centres in relation to the state of the muscle (proprioception).
- An interneuron, which affects a gamma motor neuron. This latter neuron innervates the contractile ends of the muscle spindle itself making it shorten simultaneously with the muscle fibres of the effector muscle and so ensuring that it can remain responsive to stretch. This occurs concurrently with the AMN recruitment and is termed *alpha gamma co-activation*.

Second, the efferent neuron output from the reflex arc can be modulated by neurons from higher centres. This occurs via the descending tracts (S2.14), which synapse upon the alpha motor neuron directly or indirectly via interneurons. This descending control involves altering the level of output from the AMN to the muscle by enhancing either the inhibitory or excitatory synapses as required.

REFERENCES AND FURTHER READING

Hooper SL: *Central pattern generators*, 1999, www.elsnet/elsonline/figpage/10000202html.

Kandel ER, Schwartz JH, Jessell TM: *Principles of neural science*, ed 4, New York, 2000, McGraw-Hill Health Professions Division.

Kiehn O, Butt SJ: Physiological anatomical and genetic identification of CPG neurons in the developing mammalian spinal cord, *Progress in Neurobiology* 70:347–361, 2003.

14   The descending tracts

BASIC ANATOMY AND FUNCTION OF THE MAIN DESCENDING TRACTS

The descending tracts originate from various regions of the brain stem and cerebral cortex and in the main synapse upon the alpha motor neurons (AMN) in the ventral horn of the spinal cord (S2.13). Ultimately, the AMN innervates various muscles to produce a motor contraction and achieve a motor goal. However, the descending tracts are not just a relay system as their influence via interneuron connections also gives precise control of motor output.

The descending tracts can functionally be divided into:

MEDIAL

These synapse on AMNs in a ventromedial position within the ventral horn of the grey matter of the spinal cord and innervate the muscles of the neck, trunk and proximal limb girdles.

- Medial corticospinal tract
- Reticulospinal tracts (medial and lateral)
- Vestibulospinal tracts (medial and lateral)
- Cortico-olivary tract
- Tectospinal tract.

LATERAL

These synapse on the AMNs in a dorsolateral position within the ventral horn of the grey matter of the spinal cord and innervate the muscles of the distal limbs.

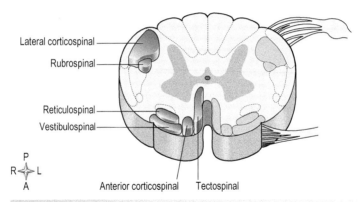

Lateral corticospinal

Rubrospinal

Reticulospinal

Vestibulospinal

P

R ✦ L

A   Anterior corticospinal   Tectospinal

Figure 14.1 A cross-section of the spinal cord showing the orientation of the main descending tracts.

- Lateral corticospinal tract
- Cortico-bulbar tract
- Cortico-rubrospinal tract.

BASIC STRUCTURE OF A DESCENDING TRACT

Most descending tracts show typical features within their anatomical structure:

A 1st order neuron with its cell body in the cerebral cortex or brain stem decussates (i.e. the neuron crosses to the opposite side of the body) and descends in the spinal cord. These neurons synapse on a 2nd order neuron

A 2nd order neuron which has its cell body in the spinal cord at the level at which it terminates/leaves the spinal cord. These neurons synapse on a 3rd order neuron

A 3rd order neuron is the AMN, with its cell body in the ventral horn of the spinal cord and which innervates a skeletal muscle.

The precise detail of each individual descending tract is beyond the scope of this book, however the function of each tract is shown in Table 14.1. Knowledge of the basic structure and anatomical orientation (Fig. 14.1) of the descending tracts, especially where each tract decussates, is important in understanding the clinical presentation of a patient with a lesion involving the spinal cord.

For example, a situation may arise whereby an incomplete spinal cord injury such as a spinal tumour may result in damage to a specific region. The consequent motor loss will be related to the particular descending tract or tracts infiltrated by the tumour (Fig. 14.1) and their specific function (Table 14.1). Depending

Table 14.1 The basic functions of the main descending tracts

Name of tract	Effector	Function
Medial corticospinal (10% of fibres)	Alpha motor neuron (AMN) of cervical and upper thoracic regions. Contralateral muscles of neck and trunk. Note: approx. 10% of fibres remain ipsilateral	Primary tract concerned with voluntary movement, specifically skilled movement
Lateral corticospinal (90% of fibres)	AMN at all levels. Contralateral distal limb (hands and feet). Note: approx. 10% of fibres remain ipsilateral	Role in fine precise movements and ability to fractionate.
Lateral/ pontine reticulospinal tracts	**Excitatory** to AMN of cervical and lumbar regions. Ipsilateral muscles of neck, trunk and proximal limb girdles	The medial and lateral tracts act together to modulate postural tone for the goal of postural stability as a background for distal movement. This is achieved by generally adjusting the level of tone and more specifically the antigravity muscles
Medial/ medullary/ reticulospinal tracts	**Inhibitory** to AMN of cervical and lumbar regions. Ipsilateral muscles of neck, trunk and proximal limb girdles	
Medial vestibulospinal tract	AMN or indirectly via interneurons of cervical and lumbar regions. Ipsilateral. Excitatory to extensor muscles and inhibitory to flexors (neck, trunk and proximal limb)	The medial and lateral vestibulospinal tracts work with the reticulospinal tracts to govern muscle tone and more specifically extensor tone related to the vestibular system's role in balance. Branches to the cranial nuclei (III, VI) control the vestibulo-ocular reflex
Lateral vestibulospinal tract	AMN or indirectly via interneuron. Ipsilateral. Excitation of extensor muscles (neck, trunk and proximal limb)	
Tectospinal tract	AMN of upper cervical segments. Contralateral neck muscles	Important in coordinating head movements with visual stimuli

Name of tract	Effector	Function
Cortico-rubrospinal tract	AMN of cervical and upper thoracic region. Contralateral. Excitatory to flexor muscles and inhibitory to extensor muscles of the upper limb	Primarily supports the the action of the corticospinal tract
Cortico-bulbar tract	Terminate at the reticular formation on the motor neurons of cranial nuclei. Ipsilateral or contralateral	Specific function relates to the function of the cranial nuclei.
Cortico-olivary tract	Cerebellum. Ipsilateral	The inferior olivary nucleus plays a role in error detection and correction for learning.

on the level of decussation, the motor loss may be contralateral or ipsilateral to the lesion.

REFERENCES AND FURTHER READING

Sherwood L: *Human physiology: from cells to systems*, ed 6, Australia, 2007, Thomson Brooks/Coles.

Snell RS: *Clinical neuroanatomy*, ed 6, Philadelphia, 2006, Lippincott Williams and Wilkins.

Tortora GJ, Derrickson B: *Essentials of anatomy and physiology*, ed 8, Hoboken, 2010, John Wiley and Sons.

CHAPTER

15

The ascending tracts

BASIC ANATOMY AND FUNCTION OF THE MAIN ASCENDING TRACTS

Basic structure of an ascending tract
Sensory receptor

BASIC ANATOMY AND FUNCTION OF THE MAIN ASCENDING TRACTS

The ascending tracts emanate from various sensory receptors in the body and convey a detailed picture of the internal and external environment to the higher centres for decision-making purposes. Some may reach the cerebral cortex and hence be of conscious awareness, while others terminate subcortically and are therefore subconscious in nature.

The main ascending tracts include:

- Spinothalamic (anterior and lateral)
- Posterior or dorsal columns
- Spinocerebellar tract (anterior and posterior).

BASIC STRUCTURE OF AN ASCENDING TRACT

As with the descending tracts, the ascending tracts have common anatomical features which generally consist of:

Sensory receptor

A 1st order neuron which is an afferent/sensory neuron in the peripheral nervous system. Its cell body is found in the dorsal root ganglion and it enters the spinal cord via the dorsal root. These neurons synapse on the 2nd order neuron

A 2nd order neuron which decussates and ascends the spinal cord in white matter to higher levels of the nervous system. These neurons synapse on the third order neuron

A 3rd order neuron usually arises from the thalamus and terminates in the somatosensory region of the parietal lobe of the cerebral cortex (S2.7). Of course those tracts that do not reach the cerebral cortex will terminate in other regions.

Knowledge of the basic structure and especially where each tract decussates is important in understanding the clinical presentation of a patient with a lesion involving the spinal cord. The precise detail of the individual ascending tracts is beyond the scope of this book, however the function of each tract is shown in Table 15.1.

Table 15.1 Basic function of the main ascending tracts

Name of tract	Function
Lateral spinothalamic	Free nerve endings provide pain and temperature information. At the level of the thalamus crude pain is perceived, however it cannot be localized (i.e. its location identified) accurately. This is only possible upon reaching the primary sensory area of the cerebral cortex (parietal lobe). The slow pain travelling in C fibres is also harder to localize than fast pain in A delta fibres.
Anterior spinothalamic	Free nerve endings provide information related to touch and pressure. At the level of the thalamus only a crude sensation is perceived. Conscious awareness is possible upon reaching the primary sensory area of the cerebral cortex (parietal lobe), however localization remains crude and discrimination of intensity is poor.
Posterior/ dorsal columns	This tract carries information related to touch, two-point discrimination and proprioception to the cerebral cortex (parietal lobe). Conscious awareness is possible upon reaching the cerebral cortex and in this case localization is more precise. Information ascending in fasciculus gracilis represents the lower limb and in fasciculus cuneatus, the upper limb.
Posterior spino- cerebellar tract	Muscle spindles and stretch receptors in the skin provide information related to position and movement of the *ipsilateral* lower limbs and trunk to the cerebellum to achieve smooth coordinated movement. As this information does not reach the cerebral cortex, it is non-conscious.
Anterior spino- cerebellar tract	Muscle spindles and stretch receptors in the skin provide information related to position and movement of the *ipsilateral* upper limbs and trunk to the cerebellum to achieve smooth coordinated movement. As this information does not reach the cerebral cortex, it is non-conscious.

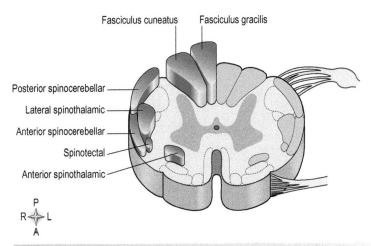

Figure 15.1 A cross-section of the spinal cord showing the orientation of the main ascending tracts.

Figure 15.1 represents the anatomical orientation of the ascending tracts within the white matter of the spinal cord. This is highly relevant in terms of a patient's clinical presentation in conditions affecting the spinal cord. For example, a situation may arise whereby an incomplete spinal cord injury due to a spinal tumour may result in damage to a specific region. The consequent sensory loss will be related to the particular ascending tract or tracts infiltrated by the tumour (Fig. 15.1) and the specific function of the tract (Table 15.1). Depending on the level of decussation the sensory loss may be contralateral or ipsilateral to the lesion.

REFERENCES AND FURTHER READING
Sherwood L: *Human physiology: from cells to systems*, ed 6, Australia, 2007, Thomson Brooks/Coles.
Snell RS: *Clinical neuroanatomy*, ed 6, Philadelphia, 2006, Lippincott Williams and Wilkins.
Tortora GJ, Derrickson B: *Essentials of anatomy and physiology*, ed 8, Hoboken, 2010, John Wiley and Sons.

SECTION 3
CLINICAL ASSESSMENT

CLINICAL ASSESSMENT

3

INTRODUCTION

Assessment is the first and arguably the most important step in the rehabilitation process, as it provides the information on which clinical reasoning will be based and upon which decision-making is reliant. The efficacy of treatment can only be as good as the assessment on which it was based (Johnson and Thompson 1996) and we only treat what it occurs to us to assess (Keshner 1991). Assessment should be an ongoing and continuous process which leads to the identification of a patient's problems, the setting of patient-centred goals and ultimately a tailor-made treatment plan for the individual (Standard 5 Core Standards of Physiotherapy Practice 2005; Edwards 2002).

By the very nature of the complexity of the nervous system, the clinical presentation of a patient with a neurological deficit is likely to be multifaceted. As such, consideration of the person as a whole during assessment and treatment is imperative to a successful outcome. Historically, biomedical models have been used as a framework for assessment. However, their focus has tended to be upon the physical consequence of the disease with little or no consideration of the psychosocial affects (Stucki and Sigl 2003).

The revised World Health Organization's (2001) publication 'International Classification of Functioning, Disability and Health' (ICF) promotes a framework for a more comprehensive assessment of the individual, providing a holistic view of health from biological, individual and social perspectives (Fig. S3.1) (Rosenbaum and Stewart 2004). This framework is relevant not only for evaluating the impact of the disease or the outcome of intervention but also for the assessment and management of limitations in function and health. The ICF framework is increasingly being

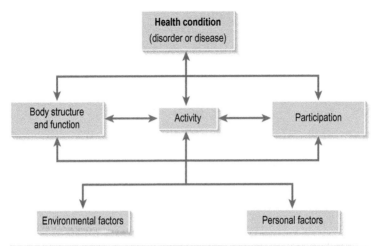

Figure S3.1 World Health Organization's International Classification of Functioning, Disability and Health (ICF).

used in clinical practice to structure the patient's problems, particularly in multidisciplinary care and for rehabilitation purposes (Stucki et al. 2002).

In the context of health, the ICF provides the following definitions (WHO 2001):

BODY STRUCTURES AND FUNCTIONS

Body functions: The physiological functions of body systems (including psychological functions)

Body structures: Anatomical parts of the body, such as organs, limbs, and their components

Impairments: Problems in body function or structure, such as a significant deviation or loss (e.g. deformity) of structures (e.g. joints) or/and functions (e.g. reduced range of movement, muscle weakness and pain). Impairments may or may not be reversible.

ACTIVITIES

Activity: Execution of a task or action by an individual (e.g. sit to stand, rolling in bed or climbing the stairs). It represents the perspective of functioning at the level of the individual.

Activity limitations: Difficulties an individual may have in executing activities.

PARTICIPATION

Participation: Involvement in a life situation (e.g. hobbies and leisure activities or employment). It represents the perspective of functioning at the level of society.

Participation restrictions: Problems an individual may experience in involvement in life situations. The limitations and restrictions are assessed against a generally accepted population norm which represents the experience of people without the specific health condition. This may include restrictions in community life, recreation and leisure, but also in walking, if walking is required to participate in a life situation.

CONTEXTUAL FACTORS

Contextual factors are those factors which constitute the complete context of an individual's life. Both contextual factors and conditions (diseases, disorders, etc.) influence disability.

Environmental factors (extrinsic influences)

This includes the physical, social, and attitudinal environment in which people live and conduct their lives. This includes the physical world and its features, other people in different relationships, roles and attitudes.

Personal factors (intrinsic influences)

The particular background of an individual's life composed of features of the individual that are not part of a health condition or health state. For example, age, gender, social status, life experiences and so on.

EVIDENCE-BASED PRACTICE IN ASSESSMENT

Although evidence of best practice related to assessment protocols is limited, there is general agreement as to the necessary tools which comprise an assessment (Standard 5, Core Standards of Physiotherapy Practice 2005). By convention, the therapist's assessment is divided into two sections: the subjective assessment and objective assessment.

The following sections, related to assessment of the neurologically impaired patient, use the ICF (WHO 2001) framework as a basis to ensure all aspects of the person are considered.

SUBJECTIVE ASSESSMENT

SUMMARY
- Informed consent
- Present complaint
- History of present complaint
  - Date of onset of the signs/symptoms
  - Progression of the condition
  - Investigation and results
  - Medical management, medical observations
  - Other management
  - Previous therapy
- Past medical history
  - Co-morbidities and other non related conditions
  - Special equipment, technology dependency
  - Previous surgery
- Drug history
  - Medication taken
- Social history
  - Personal ADL (PADL)
  - Washing, dressing, feeding/drinking, toileting
  - Domestic ADL (DADL)
  - Cooking, cleaning, shopping
- Mobility
  - General mobility
  - Walking indoors, walking outdoors
  - Stairs and steps
- Falls
- Environment
  - Home, work and hobbies
- Psychosocial
  - Personal factors
  - Lifestyle
  - Support
  - Family situation
- Record findings
- Review and note overall impression
- Plan objective assessment.

WHAT IS A SUBJECTIVE ASSESSMENT?

The subjective assessment involves gaining information about the patient and how their condition affects them as a person. Subjective information is personal to a particular patient but may originate from individuals other than the patient, e.g. relatives, carers or any member of the multidisciplinary team (MDT). This type of information may also be gathered via various communication methods, such as professional MDT notes, GP letters, a conversation with a relative or an interview/discussion with the patient.

The aim of the subjective assessment is to provide a detailed picture of how the present condition affects the patient from a holistic viewpoint. In terms of the ICF (WHO 2001) the therapist is specifically assessing:

- Activity
- Participation
- Environmental factors
- Personal factors.

WHY SHOULD I DO A SUBJECTIVE ASSESSMENT?

The reasons that the therapist needs to do a subjective assessment include:

- To identify the patient's main problems as perceived by the patient
- To assist in the setting of short and long-term goals in collaboration with the patient. Setting a goal which utilizes some functional aspects of the patient's life (e.g. work, hobbies, domestic and personal functional activities), while still incorporating therapy, is more likely to maintain motivation and interest and ultimately facilitate the patient in reaching their full potential
- To assist in the development of a relevant treatment/management plan for the individual patient
- To build a rapport with the patient.

HOW DO I DO A SUBJECTIVE ASSESSMENT?

Where do I start?

A useful exercise when preparing to carry out a subjective assessment is to reflect on the following questions:

- *What are the main categories in a subjective assessment and why do I need to ask them?*
- *Where will I get this information from? It may not always be the patient.*
- *Based upon the referral/diagnosis, what might I expect to see and hear from the patient?*
- *What may be some of the difficulties when assessing this group of patients?*
- *How will I get around these problems?*

Informed consent

To acquire informed consent is a legal, professional (Standard 2, Core Standards of Physiotherapy Practice 2005) and ethical obligation and is considered a duty that is an essential component of good clinical practice. Consent from a patient must be based on sufficient information, explained in terms the patient understands and with any risks clearly identified. The patient's choice of whether to consent must not be coerced by the therapist or any third parties, such as relatives. An individual patient must also be deemed competent to consent. That is, they are able to understand, remember, and consider the clinical information given, otherwise they may lack the autonomy to make an informed decision. The area of gaining consent and particularly judgement of competency is highly complex and the reader is referred to the Department of Health guidance (2001), along with any relevant professional body (The Chartered Society of Physiotherapy 2005).

Data collection

For details, see S3.16. It is unlikely that a subjective assessment to the detail outlined in S3.16 will be completed on the first meeting with the patient. The subjective assessment may be ongoing over several communications.

OBJECTIVE ASSESSMENT

SUMMARY
- Risk assessment
- Informed consent
- General observation (S3.17)
- Observation of *how* the patient moves during functional activities:
  - Functional activities (S3.18)
  - Gait (S3.19)
- Investigation of *why* the patient moves as they do. The therapist could include assessment of some or all of the following:
  - Postural alignment (S3.20)
  - Muscle tone (S3.21)
  - Reflexes (S3.22)
  - Sensation (S3.23)
  - Dermatomes (S3.24)
  - Trunk stability (S3.25)
  - Coordination (S3.26)
  - Vision (S3.27)
  - AROM/PROM (S3.28)
  - Pain (S3.29)
  - Strength/weakness (S3.30)
  - Myotomes (S3.31)
  - Balance (S3.32)
  - Cognition and perception (S3.33)
  - Falls (S3.34)
- Outcome measures
- Record findings
- Limitations
- Impression
- Create problem list and treatment plan.

WHAT IS AN OBJECTIVE ASSESSMENT?

An objective assessment involves the therapist gaining information related to the patient's movement disorder and functional status using measurable tools and movement analysis. In terms of the ICF (WHO 2001) the therapist is specifically assessing:

- Body structures and functions
- Activity.

In practical terms, the therapist will assess generally how the patient moves (activities) and then investigate more specifically the reasons for these movement patterns or behaviours (body structures and function). This is achieved using a combination of observation and handling skills. It is vital, where possible, to use valid and reliable outcome measures to objectify findings (Standard 6, Core Standards of Physiotherapy Practice 2005).

Assessment and treatment are often integrally linked in the assessment carried out by an experienced therapist. During the initial objective assessment, the experienced therapist may incorporate some elements of treatment, to test the potential of the patient to change. This is a skill which is only gained over time but is something for the less experienced therapist to aspire to. Of course, during ongoing treatment, the therapist should also continually re-assess to evaluate change and improvement.

WHY DO I NEED TO DO AN OBJECTIVE ASSESSMENT?

The reasons that the therapist needs to do an objective assessment include:

- Identifying the patient's movement problems and potential causes of those problems in order to appropriately focus treatment
- Providing a benchmark or baseline from which suitable short-term and long-term goals can be agreed with the patient and from which the effectiveness of treatment can be evaluated.

HOW DO I DO AN OBJECTIVE ASSESSMENT?

Where do I start?

A useful exercise when preparing to carry out an objective assessment is to reflect on the following questions:

- *What is my general impression of the patient's condition and their level of function based on the findings of my subjective assessment?*

- *What are the main categories in an objective assessment and what does each assessment tool tell me?*
- *Which assessment tools should I complete as a priority during my objective assessment? Be flexible and open minded. The initial decisions about which assessment tools to use may change as more information is gathered.*
- *What may be some of the difficulties when assessing this group of patients?*
- *How will I get around these problems?*
- *Based upon my manual handling risk assessment, do I need assistance during the objective assessment?*

Risk assessment

A manual handling risk assessment must be carried out based on the subjective information gathered. This is a legal requirement of the Manual Handling Operation Regulations (1992) and Management of the Health and Safety at Work (1999). The aim is to protect the therapist, the patient and any colleagues from potential harm. A risk assessment should consider the following:

- Task
- Individual capability
- Load
- Environment
- Other factors.

Having completed a risk assessment, the level of potential injury and the likelihood of it occurring should be evaluated. A risk management plan must then be devised and implemented. Every therapist has a legal obligation to complete and record this process.

Informed consent

To acquire informed consent is a legal, professional and ethical obligation and is considered a duty that is an essential component of good clinical practice. For further details, review the heading for informed consent under subjective assessment earlier in this section. As touch and handling techniques are necessary to carry out an objective assessment, the nature of and reasons for touch should be disclosed to the patient and if consent is given should be confirmed prior to each different technique being carried out.

Data collection

There are three main sections of a neurological assessment:

- General observation (S3.17)
- Observation of *how* the patient moves during functional activities (S3.18)
- Investigation into *why* the patient moves as they do (S3.19–34).

Note: The therapist may not be able to complete the entire objective assessment as detailed in S3.19–34. However, in an outpatient or community setting, the core of the assessment will need to be completed on the first visit in order to make a decision regarding the appropriateness of a further visit. In contrast, in an inpatient setting, the pressure to complete the whole assessment on one occasion is less and in fact may be constrained more by the patient's reduced exercise tolerance.

RECORDING

Having completed a comprehensive subjective and objective assessment, the therapist is legally responsible to keep an adequate record of the intervention, sufficient to demonstrate to a third party what, why and when the assessment was completed. The legal requirements are detailed in Standard 14 of the Core Standards of Physiotherapy (2000).

Various methods of written or electronic recording are utilized but record-keeping also incorporates video, photographs, e-mail and other media resources. The choice of recording method is one of personal taste but a commonly used system is patient-oriented medical records (POMR). This tool facilitates the problem-solving process, with the assessment forming the database on which all reasoning and decision-making is based. The particular format used varies from setting to setting but most notes related to the original database and ongoing management are written in a SOAP format. That is, the Subjective data from the patient's point of view; the Objective data acquired; the Analysis or outcome of the subjective and objective data and the action Plan. Detailed guidance on all aspects of documentation for rehabilitation can be found in Quinn and Gorden (2010).

IMPRESSION

Having reflected upon the subjective and objective assessment, it is useful to write a couple of notes (a few sentences) giving a brief overall impression of the patient. This will help guide clinical reasoning when developing the patient's problem list and treatment plan.

LIMITATIONS

As an adjunct to considering the overall impression of the patient, it is useful to note any factors that may limit the patient's progress or treatment. This may include factors such as co-morbidities and personal or environmental influences related to the ICF (WHO 2001).

CREATING A PROBLEM LIST

Using the data collected, the therapist, in collaboration with the patient, should identify the patient's main problems in the context of the whole person. A problem is defined as anything that causes concern to the patient and includes factors associated with all levels of the ICF (WHO 2001). As the patient will consider problems in a personal, environmental and social context, their perceived problems may be very different to those of a professional viewpoint.

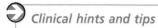

Clinical hints and tips

Developing the problem list, setting goals and treatment planning should always be done in collaboration with the patient. Patient partnership is a core standard for a physiotherapist (Standard 1). From this reasoning process, a problem list should be developed from which a structured individual treatment plan can be produced. Using the headings of the ICF may help as a guide when producing a problem list:

Body structure and function
- Decreased ROM
- Decreased muscle tone
- Low mood.

Activities
Unable to sit-to-stand.

Participation
Unable to carry out present employment as a primary school teacher.

CREATING *SMART* PATIENT-CENTRED GOALS

Goals should always be discussed and agreed with the patient. The agreed goals should then be noted in a way that fulfils the following parameters:

Specific. The goal should be focused. A goal of 'returning home' is not acceptable

Measurable. A goal could be measured using (1) a descriptive element (e.g. upright symmetrical posture); (2) by the amount of assistance/support required (e.g. with maximum assistance of 1); (3) by a time element (e.g. stand for 30 seconds); or (4) by all three

Achievable. A longer-term goal should be broken into smaller achievable parts to ensure the patient remains motivated

Repeatable/reproducible. The goal statement should be clear for any other clinician to understand and evaluate

Timed. A time should be set for the goal to be reviewed, at which point a new goal should be set or the reasons for non-achievement explained.

Short-term goals usually lie in the timeframe of 0–2 weeks, with *long-term goals* being from 2–6 weeks. However, the pathology and the individual circumstances of the patient will have an influence and need to be taken into account.

Example: short-term goal
The patient will be able to sit in an upright symmetrical posture, with stand-by assistance, for 30 seconds, in 1 week.

Example: long-term goal
The patient will be able to sit-to-stand from an armchair, weight bearing evenly through lower limbs, independently, in 3 weeks.

REFERENCES AND FURTHER READING
Chartered Society of Physiotherapy: *General principles of record keeping and access to health records PA47*, 2000. www.csp.org.uk/director/members/libraryandpublications/csppublications.cfm?item_id=74C8733B9EF7296ADB1798E7C4F1CFEA.

Chartered Society of Physiotherapy: *Consent PA60*, 2005. www.csp.org. uk/director/members/practice/informedconsent.cfm.

Core Standards of Physiotherapy Practice, 2005. www.csp.org.uk/director/members/libraryandpublications/csppublications.cfm?item_id=7 4C874E8BF4D05D6DA275134D82A846D.

Department of Health: *Reference guide to consent for examination or treatment*, London, 2001, DH.

Edwards S: *Neurological physiotherapy: a problem solving approach*, ed 2, Edinburgh, 2002, Churchill Livingstone.

Johnson J, Thompson AJ: Rehabilitation in a neuroscience centre: the role of expert assessment and selection, *British Journal of Therapy and Rehabilitation* 36:303–308, 1996.

Keshner EA: How theoretical framework biases evaluation and treatment, *Physical Therapy* 71:828, 1991.

Lord SR, Menz HB: Visual contributions to postural stability in older adults, *Gerontology* 46:306–310, 2000.

Management of Health and Safety at Work Regulations, 1999. www. opsi.gov.uk/SI/si1999/19993242.htm.

Manual Handling Operation Regulations, 1992. www.england-legislation.hmso.gov.uk/si/si1992/Uksi_19922793_en_1.htm.

Quinn L, Gorden L: *Documentation for rehabilitation: a guide to clinical decision making*, ed 2, St Louis, 2010, Saunders Elsevier.

Rosenbaum P, Stewart D: The World Health Organization International Classification of Functioning Disability and Health: a model to guide clinical thinking practice and research in the field of cerebral palsy, *Seminars in Pediatric Neurology* 111:5–10, 2004.

Stucki G, Ewert T, Cieza A: Value and application of the ICF in rehabilitation medicine, *Disability and Rehabilitation* 24:932–938, 2002.

Stucki G, Sigl T: Assessment of the impact of disease on the individual: best practice and research, *Clinical Rheumatology* 173:451–473, 2003.

WHO World Health Organization: *International Classification of Functioning Disability and Health ICF*, Geneva, 2001, World Health Organization.

Subjective assessment

Clinical hints and tips
Prior to starting the subjective assessment consider your verbal and non-verbal communication. The environment, your body language and your position in relation to the patient will influence the interaction.

PERSONAL INFORMATION

- Name
- Address
- Age
- Weight – to be used as part of a Manual Handling Risk Assessment.

>
> *Caution*
> Before you approach the patient, always double check that you have the correct patient. Patients with a neurological impairment may not always be completely reliable!

PRESENT COMPLAINT (PC)

Includes:

- The diagnosis
- The patient's main problem at the present time
- The patient's perceptions of their strengths and weaknesses
- The patient's goals and expectations of physiotherapy.

HISTORY OF PRESENT COMPLAINT (HPC)

> *Clinical hints and tips*
> Some of this information may have been collected by other professionals. To avoid asking the patient the same questions again, look at other available notes. If the multidisciplinary team uses electronic records, these should be readily available.

The therapist's questioning for this section will need to be targeted differently depending upon the type of condition (progressive or non-progressive) and the stage of the disease (acute or chronic). The important history to establish, is that leading up to the present complaint including:

DATE OF ONSET OF THE SIGNS/SYMPTOMS
This section outlines detail related to the patient's initial symptoms for the present compliant in terms of their presentation, onset time (gradual or sudden) and circumstances.

Example 1 – 1/4/09 Mr X had a left cerebrovascular accident [or CVA], while at home. Initial symptoms were slurred speech and right upper limb weakness which came on gradually. There was no loss of consciousness. Admitted to hospital via the A&E department.

Example 2 – Mr X presented with an exacerbation of lower limb spasticity, associated with MS 3/07/09. Pt referred to outpatient clinic by GP.

PROGRESSION OF THE CONDITION

The therapist should note any changes involving the initial symptoms up to the present time. In a chronic or progressive condition this may involve a long period of time. If this is the case an outline of the main history is sufficient. The history of the symptoms tells the therapist about the behaviour of the condition in the past and may therefore assist in goal setting and prediction of prognosis.

Example – Mr X was diagnosed with MS 22/11/07. Since this time he has had one exacerbation of his lower limb weakness per year, with no new additional symptoms over this period. On each occasion, a hospital admission was necessary and with medical treatment and physiotherapy he recovered sufficient mobility to return home.

Analysis – With no new neurological symptoms this may indicate that Mr X's present condition is the result of inflammation/ exacerbation of existing plaques rather than the formation of a new lesion.

INVESTIGATIONS AND RESULTS

This section should include the results of any investigations carried out which are relevant to the present condition. In a hospital setting scan results are usually found in the back of the medical notes or electronically in computerized systems. In non-hospital-based settings, the patient's GP should be able to provide these facts. Make a note of any results and the date they were undertaken (find the most recent results). This will help the therapist to start predicting the signs and symptoms likely to present and therefore plan a focused objective assessment.

Example – MRI scan showed a small infarct in the right parietal lobe 03/04/09.

MEDICAL MANAGEMENT

Note how the patient's condition has been managed by the medical team, such as neurosurgery or other medical interventions. This is relevant in all conditions and at all stages of disease and may impose limitations on the therapist's assessment and treatment.

MEDICAL OBSERVATIONS

In an acute condition or exacerbation of a chronic condition, the therapist should check the patient is medically stable before approaching to carry out the subjective assessment. Of course in a hospital-based setting with an acute admission, the therapist may continue to assess and treat patients for emergency care.

OTHER MANAGEMENT

Be aware of the management regimes implemented by other professionals in the team as they may have implication for the assessment, treatment choice and overall management.

For example, a patient being fed using percutaneous endoscopic gastrostomy (PEG) may fatigue quickly and therefore the assessment may need to be carried out over 2–3 short sessions. As receiving proper nutrition is a high priority for this patient, the assessment should try and fit around the feeding timetable. Other considerations include the patient's bladder and bowel management and communication strategies. This information should be easily accessible within the hospital setting but must also be pursued outside of this area. In the community setting, other non-healthcare agencies may be involved and their input must also be considered.

PREVIOUS THERAPY

Patients with longer-term conditions may have previously received therapy. Find out what was involved and the outcome. Their previous experience may colour the patient's expectations of the present time. Ask if they were given home exercises? Did they do them? Did it help? This may give an indication of their level of motivation. What is the patient's expectation of physiotherapy? This gives a clue about the patient's insight into their condition and if they are realistic about the future.

PAIN

Investigation of pain symptoms is important for the therapist, however it may be more convenient and less distracting for the patient to postpone this questioning until the objective assessment (S3.29).

PAST MEDICAL HISTORY (PMH)

At this stage, the therapist needs to investigate any other medical conditions and co-morbidities which may influence the patient's clinical presentation and which will need to be taken into account during assessment, treatment, goal setting and predicting the functional prognosis for the patient:

CO-MORBIDITIES
For example, mental health problems, learning disabilities, asthma, diabetes mellitus, osteoarthritis, postural hypotension and cardiac arrhythmias.

PREVIOUS SURGERY
Such as total knee replacement, laminectomy, abdominal surgery.

TECHNOLOGY DEPENDENCY
For example, a gastrostomy, nasal gastric tube, home oxygen or pacemaker.

SPECIAL EQUIPMENT
Such as suction units, special seating or walking aids.

RISK FACTORS
Risk factors related to a further neurological incident such as hypertension, raised cholesterol, diabetes mellitus, atrial fibrillation and other cardiac conditions. Note any special diet requirements and allergies.

PREVIOUS NEUROLOGICAL CONDITIONS
For example, a previous transient ischaemic attack or CVA is a strong prognostic indicator of further vascular events. Considering the amount of functional recovery from any previous events may also be useful in predicting future outcome.

DRUG HISTORY (DH)

Knowledge of the medication taken at the present time by the patient is important in terms of any relevant contraindications to therapy treatment and any related side-effects which may influence the assessment and treatment. For example, some drugs include side effects such as nausea (dantrolene), drowsiness or postural hypotension (tizanidine).

The long-term drug management of some symptoms may also result in secondary problems for the patient. For example, anti-spasmodic medications that work systemically (baclofen and tizanidine) to reduce hypertonic muscle activity are not discriminatory and therefore also affect other non-hypertonic muscles. The long-term use of these medications to reduce general muscle activity can cause underlying muscle weakness and loss of function separate to the primary condition (Dones et al. 2006).

It is also important to establish how the patient administers their medication. Can they manage themselves or do they need help? Is this assistance physical or a problem with memory/understanding? Does the administration require special/nursing skill? This latter questioning may be more relevant outside the hospital setting, but it is certainly worth considering prior to discharge from hospital.

SOCIAL HISTORY (SH)

In order to plan the objective assessment, treatment, maintain a patient's motivation and set appropriate realistic goals, the therapist needs a picture of what the patient was able to do before this incident compared with what they can do at present. The style of questioning will be dictated by many factors, including:

THE SETTING

For inpatients, some of this information can be sourced from other members of the MDT or the medical notes. In outpatients/community settings the majority of this information may need to come directly from the patient.

THE LEVEL OF FUNCTION OF THE PATIENT

It would be *inappropriate* to ask a patient who arrived at the department by bus whether he can walk to the bathroom by himself. However, if he reports the upper limb as his main problem then a detailed discussion related to how he washes, dresses and feeds himself is justified. It would also be *inappropriate* to blindly continue through the range of questions regarding mobility with a patient who is clearly severely disabled or at a very acute stage. Therefore it is necessary to be sensitive and adaptable with questioning and set the level and amount of data collected appropriately.

The following will give the therapist some idea of the type of information required:

Activities of daily living (ADL)

A detailed understanding of the patient's involvement and abilities related to personal ADL and domestic ADL will give an idea of their general level of activity and motivation. It may also highlight any issues with active/passive range of movement (ROM), strength, fine finger function, and balance which will allow the objective assessment to be more focused. Of course the ability of the patient to carry out this type of function will largely be dictated by whether their dominant hand is affected by the present condition or not.

Personal ADL (PADL)

The therapist needs to investigate both previous and present level of ability for:

Washing *Enquire do they wash in the bathroom or at the bedside?*

If they go to the bathroom do they wash at the sink or in the shower? Is the shower over the bath or can they walk in? Are there rails to assist getting into the shower? If they use the shower do they stand for the entire time or do they have a shower seat?

Do they have and can they use a bath?

When washing, how much do they do themselves? Include areas where hygiene is important such as underarms, feet and hands. Include shaving for men.

The majority of people would prefer to wash themselves; if this is not the case the therapist needs to investigate why.

Is the patient physically unable to wash? Have they taken on a sick role? Are carers taking over needlessly to save time and not allowing the patient to be independent?

This depth of questioning may appear excessive, however to ask 'Do they wash independently?' may lead to an answer of 'yes' even though what actually happens is that their carer brings a bowl of water to the bedside and they wash while sitting on the bed. This is not truly independent.

Dressing This area needs to be investigated in the same detail.

Enquire whether they can pick out their clothes from the cupboard? If not, is it because they are not physically able or do they have a perceptual/visual problem.

Does their carer lay out their clothes?

Can they do buttons or do they wear pullovers and elasticated waists to avoid the problem? Can they do up shoe laces? Can women manage a bra and men manage a tie?

Feeding/drinking In situations where no speech and language therapy (SALT) assessment has been carried out, ask about the ability to eat and drink. Most importantly:

Do they have difficulty swallowing? Do they cough or choke after eating or drinking? If a problem is identified in this area, that is not currently being managed, then it is the therapist's responsibility to make a referral to SALT so that the patient can be properly assessed. In this case, a physiotherapy respiratory assessment will also be indicated.

Investigation related to the act of eating/drinking is also necessary. *Can they use a knife and fork?* Can they cut up their own food? Can they transfer food from plate to mouth successfully?

Toileting Information regarding continence of bladder and bowel should already be available in a hospital setting. However, if a problem is identified that is not being managed, questioning should be discrete and sensitive followed by a referral to the relevant professional. It is always worth checking where incontinence is highlighted, whether the patient has accidents because they simply cannot get to the toilet quick enough. A brief enquiry related to the ability to remove the relevant clothes for toileting and carry out their own hygiene post-toileting may also be informative.

Domestic ADL (DADL)

Questioning related to the present level of ability in these activities will not be relevant in a hospital setting. However, an understanding of the patient's previous levels, to which they may strive, is appropriate. Where required investigate both previous and present levels for:

Cooking *Did they do the cooking before this incident?*

What can they manage now and how do they do it? For example, can they pick up a full kettle or saucepan? Can they make themselves a sandwich? Can they prepare a proper meal or do they use microwave meals?

Cleaning *Did they do the cleaning before this incident?*

What can they manage now and how do they do it? For example, can they do the hoovering? Can they manage light dusting? Can they make the bed or iron clothes?

Shopping *Did they do the shopping before this incident?* Can they manage shopping at the local shop? Can they manage at a supermarket? The latter two situations have very different physical demands. If they do not go out shopping, is it related to a physical constraint or is it because they do not want to be seen in public?

MOBILITY

Note that the patient's mobility may change at different times of the day. This could relate to factors such as general fatigue, other non-related conditions, poor motivation or medications but when identified, should be investigated thoroughly. Enquire about these different aspects of mobility prior to the present condition and at present:

General mobility

This will include examples of all transfers, such as sitting to standing, sitting to lying, rolling, etc. When possible, ask the patient about these transfers in functionally relevant circumstances. For example, can they manage to get from lying to sitting over the edge of the bed in the morning? Can they stand up from the toilet/low sofa/armchair? These situations have different demands.

Walking indoors

How far can they walk indoors?

Are they independent? Do they use a walking aid? Do they hold onto the furniture? This is extremely unsafe. Do they need assistance from a relative or carer? If yes, how much assistance? Is help required to stand up or while walking?

Walking outdoors

How far can they walk outdoors?

Are they independent? Do they need a walking aid and/or assistance? How do they cope with slopes (up and down), rough ground, kerb stones, other pedestrians?

Stairs and steps

Are they independent? Do they use the hand rails? Do they use a walking aid and/or need assistance.

Falls

The National Institute for Clinical Excellence (NICE) guidelines for falls (2004) recommend that older people be asked *routinely* whether they have fallen in the past year and the frequency, context and characteristics of the fall(s). When the individual reports recurrent falls within the year, the NICE guidance is that they should be offered a multifactorial falls risk assessment (S3.34).

Other

Do they do any form of exercise at home? What type? How often? Do they feel it benefits them and if so how? How do they cope walking in unfamiliar surroundings? Do they drive, ride a bicycle or use public transport?

 Clinical hints and tips

An easy way to gain the majority of this social history (as long as conversation is guided) is to ask the patient to talk through a normal day. This also provides insight into the patient's general activity levels, motivation and how much responsibility the patient takes for themselves.

ENVIRONMENT

A detailed investigation around this topic is important in all areas but especially so in an outpatient and community setting and as part of discharge planning in the hospital setting. Although in some settings a home visit will be carried out prior to discharge, it is still useful to gain an overview of the patient's environment to enable the therapist to give a personal focus to goals and treatment.

Do they live in a house, bungalow, flat, caravan?

Is access to the home manageable? Are there any steps outside? Is there a handrail on the steps/stairs? Which side is it on?

Ask about the general layout of their home? Is there a bathroom downstairs?

Is the area they live in urban/rural, hilly or flat? If relevant, make similar enquiries related to work and any separate venues used to pursue hobbies?

If problems related to the housing environment are identified and are not being managed, then the therapist is responsible for a referral to the appropriate agency (Occupational Therapy, Social Services, etc.).

PSYCHOSOCIAL

Psychosocial factors play an important part in the physical, cognitive and emotional wellbeing of the patient. However, sensitive questioning may be required and where issues arise that are outside the therapist's area of competency, a referral to the appropriate professional is essential. The therapist should consider the following:

Personal factors

These maybe reported more frequently by close friends and relatives. For example, lack of confidence, low self-esteem, depression, anxiety, stress, challenging behaviour and lack of motivation. A sudden change in the role of the patient in relation to the family can cause great upheaval and stress for all and can have serious financial implications.

Life style This includes:

Occupation: Is the patient retired, employed or self-employed? What does the job entail? Ask for detail if it is not something obvious. This will be useful in setting appropriate goals and can be used as part of treatment.

Hobbies, recreational activities and sport: Question as for occupation.

Education: Does the patient attend school, further or higher education, or are they an adult learner?

Support Questioning should incorporate:

Personal support: Who is local and supportive of the patient's needs – family, friends, colleagues or dependants? What commitments and pressures do these people have? What perceptions and expectations do these individuals have? Their attitudes may facilitate or limit the patient's progress.

Finances: Is the patient financially independent/dependent? Are they receiving any sort of benefit (Disability Living Allowance, Employment/Pensions/Housing benefit)?

Family situation Does the patient live alone, married or have children? What is the general situation of the patient's family – culture, religion and language? Are they categorized as homeless, refugee, asylum seekers, vulnerable, single parents?

PLANNING THE OBJECTIVE ASSESSMENT

The role of the therapist is to interpret the information that the patient relates to them in order to plan the objective assessment and implement patient-centred goals and effective treatment. This requires clinical analysis of the subjective assessment in terms of:

- Which information is clinically relevant and which is not
- Which functions are difficult for the patient and whether there are any common factors influencing them all. These functions

then need to be broken down to analyse the likely joint movements, muscle actions and motor control aspects. From this basic knowledge, the therapist can begin to reason the potential causes of the patient's difficulties based on the presenting pathology.

Following this analysis, the therapist should be confident to start making decisions to ensure that the objective assessment is more focused. This skill takes time to develop but becomes easier with experience.

REFERENCE

Dones I, Nazzi V, Tringali G, et al. Cautious use of intrathecal baclofen in walking spastic patients: results on long-term follow-up, *Neuromodulation* 9(2):87–93, 2006.

17

Objective assessment (general observation)

VISION

HEARING

COMMUNICATION

COGNITION AND PERCEPTION

GENERAL APPEARANCE

BEHAVIOUR

EXERCISE TOLERANCE

These signs will primarily be observed as the patient enters the department, or during the subjective and objective assessments. They *may not* be formally assessed by the therapist but may require referral to another professional as appropriate.

VISION

Does the patient wear glasses? What do they wear them for? Will they need them on for therapy? When was their last eye check? Often individuals have retained old glasses that are now unsuitable.

HEARING

This will have been apparent during the subjective assessment. Do they wear a hearing aid? Is it switched on? Is it clogged with wax? If they are not wearing one, should they be? Be sensitive when questioning the patient, poor concentration/attention may present similarly.

COMMUNICATION

Does the patient have a problem expressing her/himself or understanding your requests? This could be related to the points above or a deficit of speech or cognition.

COGNITION AND PERCEPTION

Does the patient have trouble concentrating during the assessment? Do they have difficulty understanding instructions or solving a simple problem? Do they have difficulty dressing or undressing? Do they perform tasks in the wrong order or miss out elements of the task?

Any cognitive and perceptual deficit will have implications for your communication with the patient and hence the success of any interaction. S3.33 may give the therapist some insight into the cause of these presentations.

GENERAL APPEARANCE

Does the patient appear unkempt? This may indicate that the patient is not coping at home. Sensitive questioning may be required but this is not essential immediately. Presentation of certain postures may also be indicative of a clinical pathology. For example, a slouched, flexed posture in combination with other signs and symptoms may suggest clinical depression.

BEHAVIOUR

Does the patient behave inappropriately (physically or verbally)? Are they inappropriately euphoric or tearful? Are they aggressive? Any aggressive behaviour needs to be highlighted to the rest of the multidisciplinary team (MDT) and a risk assessment carried out. These presentations could indicate damage to the frontal lobe, limbic system or may reflect a mental health problem. As such differential diagnosis is crucial, these complex presentations require a comprehensive assessment by a competent professional.

EXERCISE TOLERANCE

Do they fatigue very quickly on activity? Do they become breathless?

18 Objective assessment (functional assessment)

OBSERVATION OF HOW THE PATIENT MOVES	The quality of performance/ movement analysis
Patient	
Therapist	
Functional ability	ANALYSIS

OBSERVATION OF HOW THE PATIENT MOVES

This part of the assessment can be completed while the patient carries out *a functional transfer* such as rolling, sitting to lying, lying to sitting, sitting to standing, standing to sitting, walking indoors/outdoors, stairs, running. However, it is equally useful to assess the patient's movement during *functional activities*, for example, dressing/undressing, reach and grasp, writing their name, etc.

PATIENT

The function/s chosen to observe will depend on the patient's ability. For example, if the patient is unable to move out of bed, then start your assessment with bed mobility. On the other hand, if the patient walks into the department, then the assessment will be set at a higher level of function.

Note: If the patient is able to walk, then the therapist will also need to complete a full gait analysis (S3.19).

THERAPIST

The aim of observing function is to identify any movement abnormalities and as such, the patient must be physically challenged. However, care should be taken not to fatigue the patient. Ultimately, all transfers will need to be assessed for the therapist to gain a full understanding of functional ability.

While the patient performs the function the therapist needs to note:

Functional ability

That is, how successful the patient is and what assistance they require completing the task. For example, the patient is independent sitting to standing *or* the patient needs minimal assistance of 1 from lying to sitting.

The quality of performance/movement analysis

The therapist also needs to analyse how they perform the function. In essence this is movement analysis. At this point the therapist is trying to identify any deviations from the normal limits of efficient movement and not necessarily the underlying cause of the deviations. This demands the therapist has a good understanding of the requirements of the task and may require the inexperienced therapist to carry out a task analysis prior to observing the patient. The task analysis should be considered in relation to the wide variation of normal presentations possible. A good understanding of basic biomechanical principles will also facilitate the therapist's reasoning during this process.

Normal requirements of the task   To facilitate this process, the therapist may choose to base their analysis on the following basic structure:

- Start position – in relation to joint angles
- Finish position – in relation to joint angles
- Muscle action – in terms of how the individual moves from start to finish position. Consider:
  - Which muscles are required
  - The function of the muscle during the task (agonist, antagonist, synergist)
  - Type of muscle contraction (eccentric, isometric, concentric)
  - Range of the muscle work (inner, middle, outer).

 Caution

The range of strategies implemented within normal limits of efficient movement (i.e. a healthy population) will be wide ranging. Therefore, when setting the normal requirements of any task the therapist should be cautious and flexible in approach.

Patient observation Based on the analysis of the normal task requirements the therapist should record any deviations from their expectation of what is efficient movement. However they should also note the presentation of any of the following:

- General postural alignment
  Are there any obvious asymmetries? Does the movement adhere to biomechanical principles? Altered alignment could indicate: (1) instability due to hypotonia or weakness; (2) a restriction due to hypertonia, soft tissue shortening or pain, or (3) altered sensation. More detailed postural alignment and differential diagnosis of cause should be investigated later in the assessment.
- Quality of movement
  Is the movement smooth, coordinated, well timed, effortless? Poor quality movement could result from a motor or sensory impairment or a problem with integration. Ataxia (S3.26) also manifests as incoordinated movement of the limbs or trunk but is due to a dysfunction of the cerebellum (S2.12).
- Compensations
  Do they use any trick movements during functional activities? Is the movement successful in achieving the motor goal? Compensation is defined as a behavioural substitution adopted to complete a task (Shumway-Cook and Woollacott 2007). As motor control is goal orientated, a successful compensatory movement may result in the central nervous system adopting this strategy in the long term rather than finding other solutions. This may limit the individual from recovering to their full potential (Cristea and Levin 2000). While it is acknowledged that compensations also occur within a healthy population, it is this lack of choice of movement solutions in neurologically impaired patients that limits their function (Raine et al. 2009). Therefore perhaps therapy should be aimed at facilitating a choice of compensations or modifying the most inefficient ones.
- Patterns of movement
  Do they use normal movement patterns? Do they use gross movement patterns? This is due to the inability to fractionate or break up a basic pattern of movement in order to make it functional. Fractionation is defined as the ability to move a single joint without simultaneously moving other joints (Shumway-Cook and Woollacott 2007). All tasks require a combination of muscle synergies. For example, the task of reaching requires

shoulder flexion, elbow and wrist extension with finger flexion to grip. Therefore, an individual who uses a gross pattern involving flexion at all joints will be ineffective in achieving their goal. This is one of the signs of spasticity (S3.21).

- Involuntary movements

  Do they present with dystonia? Dystonia is a syndrome character- ized by abnormal, sustained muscle contractions often resulting in persistent abnormal postures at the extremes of movement range. The movements are often twisting and range in speed and amplitude. Abnormal co-contraction is common and the contractions often elicit pain. Dystonia is associated with lesions of the basal ganglia (S2.11), particu- larly the indirect pathway of the putamen nucleus. However, there are several subtypes which may vary in cause.

  Do they present with athetoid movements? Athetoid movements are slow writhing twisting movements of small amplitude primarily involving the upper limb.

  Do they present with choreiform movements? Choreiform move- ments are rapid, jerky movements often of large amplitude. This presentation is observed in Huntington's chorea and caused by a lesion of the basal ganglia (indirect pathway).

  Do they present with clonus? Clonus is most commonly seen at the ankle and presents as a rhythmic oscillation between plantar flexion and dorsiflexion. This occurs when a brief stretch of the plantar flexor muscle occurs and the tension is maintained, e.g. when placing the affected lower limb of a patient up onto the footplate of a wheelchair.

  Do they present with any associated reactions (ARs)? An AR is a temporary involuntary movement primarily involving the upper limb. The initiating triggers are widely variable and individual to the patient but can include increased effort during movement (Bhakta et al. 2001), muscular instability, yawning, coughing, pain, fear, urinary tract infection. Little evidence exists as to the underlying cause of these reactions but the time delay in onset after the original lesion seems to implicate maladaptive changes which lead to a reduced ability to inhibit unwanted movement. This is one of the signs of spasticity (S3.21). When associated reactions are evident, it is important that the therapist records:

  - *When the AR occurs precisely,* e.g. during mid-stance of the right lower limb
  - *The excursion of the movement,* e.g. elbow flexion occurs to a maximum of 90°

- *The pattern of the movement*, e.g. elbow flexion with forearm pronation and some finger flexion
- *How long the AR remains*, e.g. the upper limb immediately returns to normal when the patient stops walking. There is no AR in standing.

This information will provide clues as to any movement trigger that exists, e.g. an area of instability or poor balance.

- Active range of movement (AROM)
  Are there any obvious limitations in AROM? (S3.28), e.g. taking off a jacket or jumper requires good AROM of the shoulder and trunk in certain directions. Any limitation may be a result of soft tissue shortening, muscle weakness (S3.30), pain (S3.29), altered sensation (S3.23) or altered muscle tone (S3.21)
- Balance
  Do they lose balance or stumble during any activity? (S3.32, 34). This may be a direct result of a deficit affecting the balance systems (vestibular system/vision/proprioception) or a functional consequence of various other symptoms, such as poor trunk stability, altered muscle tone or sensation.
- Lack of confidence
  Do they appear anxious during movement? Patients who are fearful of movement will often limit their function. This can be a result of many factors including previous falls.
- Exercise tolerance
  Do they fatigue very quickly on activity? Do they become breathless?

ANALYSIS

Having completed the observation of the patient during a functional activity and noted any deviations, the therapist can begin to reason what the potential causes of the dysfunction could be based upon the task requirements. The hypothesis generated will need to be tested and confirmed using the specific assessment tools (S3.19–34).

REFERENCES

Bhakta BB, Cozens JA, Chamberlain MA, et al. Quantifying associated reactions in the paretic arm in stroke and their relationship to spasticity, *Clinical Rehabilitation* 15:195–206, 2001.

Cristea MC, Levin MF: Compensatory strategies for reaching in stroke, *Brain* 123:940–953, 2000.

Raine S, Meadows L, Lynch-Ellerington M: *Bobath concept: theory and clinical practice in neurological rehabilitation*, Oxford, 2009, Wiley-Blackwell.

Shumway-Cook A, Woollacott MH: *Motor control: translating research into clinical practice*, ed 3, Philadelphia, 2007, Lippincott Williams and Wilkins.

Gait

WHAT IS GAIT?

Gait is a highly energy efficient method of locomotion necessary for most daily activities. It involves rhythmical, reciprocal movements of the lower limbs and in terms of biomechanics reflects a destabilizing phase followed by a stabilizing phase (Magee 2006). Commonly, the gait cycle is described in terms of a stance phase (approximately 60% of time) and a swing phase (approximately 40%). The tasks involved in gait include: progression within space but also the achievement of a stable alternating one leg stand and postural stability to maintain an upright stance during all phases. Although for the majority of time gait is automatic, requiring no conscious thought, it actually comprises complex patterns of movement involving the whole body. The rhythmic, repetitive components of gait are thought to be initiated and controlled by central pattern generators within the spinal cord (S2.13). However, when changes in the internal and external environment occur, higher level centres are required to integrate and coordinate the motor response. Therefore, if the central nervous system is damaged the functional ability of a patient to walk is likely to be impaired.

The normal gait cycle is defined as the sequence of motions between two consecutive contacts of the same foot, e.g. heel strike of the left foot to heel strike of the left foot. Stance phase involves heel strike to toe off of the same lower limb (LL), while swing phase includes an initial acceleration phase through to a terminal deceleration phase. An understanding of the normal gait cycle (Figs 19.1, 19.2) and its biomechanics in terms of joint angles and muscle activity is vital to completing a sound assessment, with insufficient knowledge leading to incorrect analysis. A detailed description of normal gait is beyond the scope of this text, however a brief overview of the mechanics of the lower limb is noted

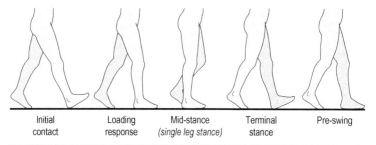

| Initial contact | Loading response | Mid-stance *(single leg stance)* | Terminal stance | Pre-swing |

Figure 19.1 Main components of stance phase of the gait cycle.

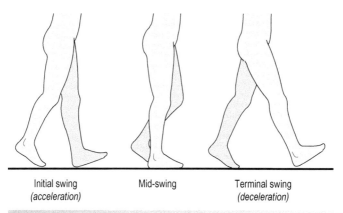

| Initial swing *(acceleration)* | Mid-swing | Terminal swing *(deceleration)* |

Figure 19.2 Main components of swing phase of the gait cycle.

below. It should be stressed that all the elements described are integrated in real-time during gait and the therapist should not forget to consider the head/neck, trunk and upper limbs, which are integral in efficient gait.

STANCE PHASE (FIG. 19.1)

Ankle: Dorsiflexion for heel strike, eccentric control of dorsiflexion to gain flat foot, dorsiflexion to achieve mid-stance and plantarflexion for push off

Knee: Slight knee flexion at heel strike (acting as a shock absorber), full extension at mid-stance and slight flexion in preparation for swing phase

Hip: Flexion at heel strike followed by extension and adduction to gain mid-stance and weight transfer. Full hip extension at the end of stance phase just prior to push off

Pelvis: Lateral shift towards stance, lower limb.

SWING PHASE (FIG. 19.2)

Ankle: Dorsiflexion at toe off and maintained in preparation for heel strike

Knee: Flexion to shorten the lower limb for ground clearance during swing. Knee extension in preparation for heel strike

Hip: Flexion to initiate acceleration of lower limb at toe off in swing and eccentric control of flexion to decelerate in preparation for heel strike

Pelvis: Slight drop and rotation forward on swing lower limb side at toe off.

WHY DO I NEED TO ASSESS GAIT?

Gait dysfunction is common in neurologically impaired patients and can occur from a myriad of different signs and symptoms associated with the pathology. The factors influencing gait may be a direct result of the pathology such as changes in muscle tone, sensation or cognitive and perceptual deficits or due to secondary disuse and inactivity. For example, muscle weakness, alteration of soft tissue extensibility, reduced exercise tolerance or reduced confidence. (For more detail on how specific impairments affect gait, the reader is referred to Chapter 14 in Shumway-Cook and Woollacott 2007).

Dysfunction of gait is one of the earliest and commonest problems reported by patients, with the inability to move around the environment being stated as a critical factor in individuals becoming more dependent and suffering a reduced quality of life. The ability to walk is often, but not always, the goal most eagerly pursued by patients.

Therefore, a detailed assessment of a patient's gait is essential in order to set a benchmark from which appropriate goals can be set and an efficient gait pattern achieved. A more efficient gait is likely to be more energy efficient and safer in terms of falling. It may also prevent or at least limit secondary musculoskeletal complications.

HOW DO I DO GAIT ANALYSIS?

OBSERVATION

Gait analysis may be carried out in many ways and the method chosen should be based on what the individual therapist finds most helpful. One method is highlighted below.

Patient

Initially the therapist needs to establish how the patient chooses to move without any intervention.

Therapist

1. Sufficient assistance must be given during the assessment to ensure the safety of the patient.
2. The therapist should observe the gait from all directions (front, behind and side) paying attention to each of the main body segments, head/neck, shoulder complex, upper limb, trunk, pelvis, hip and lower limb.
3. These body segments are then observed during one phase of gait at a time. For example, watch the whole body during stance phase of the left lower limb (incorporating right lower limb swing phase) and then repeat the observation during right lower limb stance phase (incorporating left lower limb swing phase).

Clinical hints and tips

Gait analysis may take some time for the inexperienced therapist and as such the exercise tolerance of the patient may be a limiting factor. Video-recording the patient gives the therapist an opportunity to review the gait without fatiguing the patient.

4. The therapist should observe each body segment in terms of:
   General alignment of body segments
   Changes to normal gait cycle, including omissions from and alterations in sequence and timing. For example, no heel strike, no terminal hip extension, decreased stride length, increased foot angle or uncontrolled foot placement
   Abnormal movements, e.g. associated reactions in the upper limb (S3.18). Again it is important to note the timing of these reactions for accurate analysis
   Increased effort
   Lack of confidence
   Altered balance

5. The therapist should, where appropriate, assess the patient walking in different directions (forwards, backwards, sideways, turning) and in different contexts (indoors on various surfaces and outdoors on uneven surfaces).

6. Foot and ankle: The foot provides the main source by which muscle recruitment is adapted during gait (Holland and Lynch-Ellerington 2009). Therefore the mobility of the foot and ankle joints and the stability gained from intrinsic muscles may require particular attention. This may be carried out later in the objective assessment.

RECORDING

A text description of the deficits of gait may be structured under the relevant phase of gait or related to body segments. The example below relates to Figure 19.3.

Example

Pt X walks independently with a walking stick carried in the right hand. Using a reciprocal pattern with a 3-point gait.

During left stance phase/right swing phase:

Head and neck: left side flexed with slight right rotation
Shoulder complex: left side rotated backwards
Trunk: left side rotated backwards
UL, left: pt exhibits an associated reaction (glenohumeral joint extended with elbow flexed to 90°, forearm supination and finger flexion). This associated reaction is increased during left stance and decreases during right stance
UL, right: pt tends to hold walking stick far out to the right
Pelvis: left side rotated backwards

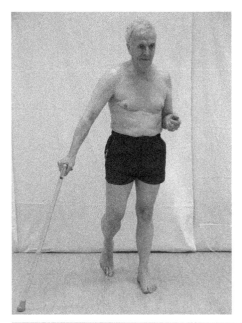

Figure 19.3 Gait analysis of left stance phase.

Hip, left: slight medial rotation. Pt unable to achieve terminal extension
Hip, right: slight abduction and external rotation
Ankle/Foot, left: unable to gain flat foot
Ankle/foot, right: pt tends to take a quick short step through.

ANALYSIS

In terms of clinical reasoning, the gait analysis itself may allow the therapist to produce a hypothesis as to the causes of any deviation from normal, however this will need to be tested and confirmed in Part 3 of the objective assessment (S3.20–34).

In the above example, the gait analysis may lead the therapist to suspect (1) an area of instability (trunk, hip/pelvis) on the left side which leads the patient to lack confidence or the ability to transfer weight over the affected left lower limb and achieve terminal hip extension. The associated reaction could also reflect the instability acting as a balance mechanism for an alignment that lacks equilibrium. Or (2) the foot/ankle may also be causal as the inability to gain flat foot could also produce the malalignments described above.

OUTCOME MEASURES

RESEARCH

In recent years technology has developed high quality accurate measurement tools in relation to kinematic or kinetic data by which any movement can be objectively analysed. The use of this technology improves the quality and rigour of gait analysis for the assessment.

- Electromyography (EMG)
- SiliconCOACH Pro version 6.0 program (2004)
- VICON digital optical motion capture
- Force platform.

CLINICAL

Various outcome measures exist to measure different quantitative aspects of gait and it is important that the therapist understands what is being measured by these measures and then selects one that is appropriate to need.

- 10-metre timed – walk speed
- 6-minute walk – endurance
- Timed get up and go – balance and integration into function
- Step count (number of steps over a set distance)
- Cadence (number of steps per minute).

REFERENCES AND FURTHER READING

Holland A, Lynch-Ellerington M: The control of locomotion. In Raine S, Meadows L, Lynch-Ellerington M, editors: *Bobath concept: theory and clinical practice in neurological rehabilitation*, Oxford, 2009, Wiley-Blackwell.

Magee DJ: *Orthopaedic physical assessment*, ed 4, Canada, 2006, Elsevier Sciences.

Moore S, Schurr K, Wales A, et al: Observation and analysis of hemiplegic gait: stance phase, *Australian Journal of Physiotherapy* 39:259–267, 1993.

Moore S, Schurr K, Wales A, et al: Observation and analysis of hemiplegic gait: swing phase, *Australian Journal of Physiotherapy* 39:271–278, 1993.

Shumway-Cook A, Woollacott MH: *Motor control: translating research into clinical practice*, ed 3, Philadelphia, 2007, Lippincott Williams and Wilkins.

SiliconCOACH: *SiliconCOACH Coaching solutions for a digital age* [online]. New Zealand, 2004. www.siliconcoach.com (Accessed 1 September 2006).

Postural alignment 20

WHAT IS POSTURAL ALIGNMENT?

Postural alignment refers to the relationship between body segments and in basic terms refers to the structure of the musculoskeletal system, bones, joints and muscles. The alignment of the musculoskeletal system, within normal limits, is important in terms of minimizing stresses on soft tissue, minimizing muscle effort and providing sensory information to the centres involved in motor control (the control of movement). Hence, the musculoskeletal alignment plays a significant role in facilitating efficient movement during functional activities (Lennon 2003; Mayston 2000a,b; Carr and Shepherd 2003).

The importance of sensory feedback to successful motor control is well established (Kandel et al. 2000), with all decisions made by the nervous system being based upon the sensory feed forward/ feedback it receives. A successful outcome is therefore reliant upon receiving sufficient accurate sensory information, a large amount of which comes from the somatosensory receptors (S3.23) embedded in the musculoskeletal system. In the main, this information relates to proprioception (S3.23), joint and muscle position and movement sense. Therefore it is the alignment of the musculoskeletal system which informs the nervous system of its present state for the planning of movement and also its ongoing state during movement when outcome can be monitored.

The alignment of body segments is therefore critical in both posture (arrested movement) and movement itself. The relationship between posture and movement can be viewed as integral in terms of body segment alignment with similar patterns or strategies observed in both. To appreciate any deviations from a normal range, the therapist requires knowledge of the normal parameters of posture and movement patterns and the range of normal presentations.

WHY DO I NEED TO ASSESS POSTURAL ALIGNMENT?

A deviation from the most efficient alignment of the musculoskeletal system can occur as a direct effect of various neurological impairments, e.g. as a result of hypertonia, hypotonia (S3.21); pain (S3.29); weakness (S3.30) or altered sensation (S3.23). The malalignment of one body segment may also produce further deviations from normal range in other segments. For example, hypotonia involving the shoulder complex will directly result in reduced stability at the glenohumeral joint and possibly a subluxation. However, the changes in biomechanics will also immediately influence the alignment of both the upper limbs and the trunk as the patient finds strategies to compensate and remain balanced. The extra effort required to move and the stresses on soft tissue may later produce pain which will further limit the biomechanics of the movement. Over time, soft tissue adaptation occurs and the new compensatory strategies become learned via the physiological processes of neuroplasticity (Ungerleider et al. 2002; Marrone 2007).

Following a change in the musculoskeletal alignment of a body, there is a corresponding change in the somatosensory feedback to the nervous system. In the case of patients with a neurological deficit, they may be further disadvantaged by having a direct lesion involving the sensory system which may limit the *amount* and *accuracy* of the feedback. Potentially this could lead to an inaccurate motor plan being implemented and ultimately an inefficient, unsuccessful movement.

In terms of treatment, the therapist will aim to facilitate a musculoskeletal alignment that is within normal limits for both posture and movement.

HOW DO I ASSESS POSTURAL ALIGNMENT?

OBSERVATION

As the patterns of musculoskeletal alignment are similar for posture and movement, the initial assessment can be carried out in a static posture. The assessment of alignment during movement is covered in the second part of the objective assessment section whereby the therapist performs a movement analysis of a functional task (S3.18).

Patient

The posture chosen will vary according to the patient's ability. For example, for a patient recently admitted with no sitting balance it will be safer in a supported sitting or supine position.

Clinical hints and tips

Keep in mind that until you have more experience the process may take some time and sitting or standing for a long period may be uncomfortable for some people.

The same malalignments can often be observed in any posture, but will be more pronounced when the patient is in a more challenging posture, such as sitting and standing.

Therapist

1. Where possible each of the main joints should be observed individually. This is necessary in order to establish the *specific* location of any deviation. For example, recording protraction at the shoulder complex is insufficient, as protraction involves a combination of movements at the glenohumeral joint, sternoclavicular and acromioclavicular joint and scapulothoracic joint. In order to target treatment effectively, the alignment of each should be evaluated.

Caution
Do not to start analysing the data until you have recorded all your findings from the individual body segments. You may start to question correctly that a deviation in one segment is occurring because of the influence of another, however waiting until the full picture is available will improve your overall analysis and conclusions.

2. The therapist should observe the alignment of all the body segments from all directions (in front, behind and from the side) taking into account all aspects of the segment orientation (anterior/posterior, superior/inferior, medial/lateral and rotation). Observing from different directions will allow the therapist to confirm the location of a deviation and its orientation/relationship with other segments.

3. The therapist may gain clues related to any deviation by observing or palpating:
   - Skin creases
   - Bony points
   - Joint lines
   - Weight bearing status
   - Adjacent muscle activity.

Clinical hints and tips
Although this assessment is primarily achieved via observation, the accuracy will depend upon your palpation of bony points to establish exactly the location and orientation of a body segment.

4. The orientation of each segment can be noted using descriptors based on the physiological movements possible at the joint. For example, when evaluating the hip joint, the descriptors available would be flexion, extension, abduction, adduction, medial and lateral rotation.
   Is the segment orientated in a neutral position?
   Is the segment symmetrical in relation to a bilateral structure (e.g. the scapulas), to a midline structure (e.g. spinous processes) and to structures above and below?

Is the posture itself having any influence on segment alignment? Certain postures will impose deviations and should be recorded (e.g. hip flexion in sitting) but should not influence analysis. However, if the response bilaterally is not symmetrical (e.g. left hip is externally rotated and abducted in relation to the right), then further analysis is recommended.

RECORDING

When recording the findings there are a few viable options to choose from. Namely:

- Body chart (see Fig. 20.3). Remember that when using a body chart include a key to identify the symbols used and before adding data to the chart, label left and right on each figure to avoid mistakes
- Text description (Table 20.1)
- Table (Table 20.2).

Example

The following examples relate to Figures 20.1 and 20.2.

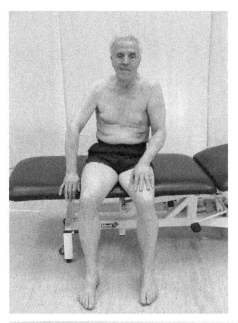

Figure 20.1 Anterior view of patient X.

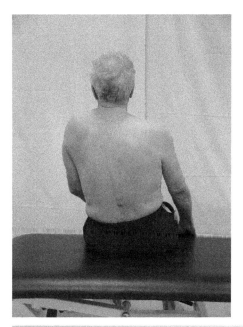

Figure 20.2 Posterior view of patient X.

Table 20.1 Text description of the postural alignment assessment of patient X (pt X)

Patient sitting:
   The trunk is left side flexed, with the left side rotated forward and right side rotated backwards. The right side of the trunk appears under active.
   The right scapula is abducted, depressed and lat. rotated with under activity around the medial border. The left scapula is elevated and appears to have overactive elevators.
   Right UL has a predominance of flexor activity.
   The right side of the pelvis is rotated backwards and the right hip is abducted and externally rotated with under activity surrounding the hip.
   The patient is primarily weight bearing through the left side.

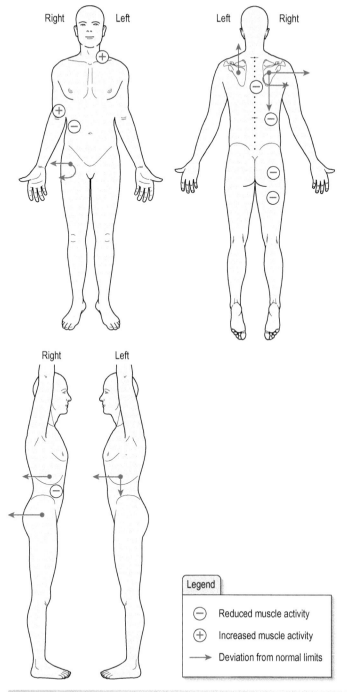

Figure 20.3 Example of body chart recording (postural alignment).

Table 20.2 Table representation of the postural alignment assessment of patient X (pt X)

Body segment	Malalignments noted		
Head/neck	Nil of note		
Trunk	Side flexion (Left)	Rotation (Left forward)	Rotation (Right backward)
	Right side under active		
Scapula	Right depressed/Abd/Lat rotated/Left elevated		
	Right scapula under active (med border)/Left scapula over active elevators		
GH joint	Predominance of flexor over activity		
Pelvis	Right side rotated backwards		
Hip	Right side Abd/Lat rotated		
	Underactive around hip		
Weight bearing	Primarily over left side		

ANALYSIS

Having completed the assessment, the therapist should have identified any deviations outside the normal limits expected. During the analysis of this data, the therapist should start to hypothesize the relationship between any deviations presented and begin to try and predict which may be causal and which may be a compensation in response. Gathering more information from the remaining objective assessment tools will be necessary before the reason for the deviations can be established.

Example

The body chart (Fig. 20.3) represents patient X shown in Figures 20.1 and 20.2 who has suffered a right hemiplegia. Following analysis of all the objective markers and examination of the body chart the following is hypothesized. The right pelvis, hip, trunk and shoulder complex are seen to be rotated backwards probably due to hypotonia. In response, the patient works harder with the left side, especially the shoulder complex (elevation) and forward trunk rotation in an attempt to maintain an upright posture against gravity. The latter is a normal response to the deviation imposed by the hypotonia on the right. Therefore treatment would be most effective aimed at the hypotonia with the assumption that the compensatory activity would then no longer be required.

OUTCOME MEASURES

RESEARCH

Objective tools capable of measuring the alignment of structures of the musculoskeletal system include:

- Analysis of digital video by SiliconCOACH Pro version 6.0 program (2004) or Matlab program 7.0 (Mathworks) software
- VICON digital optical motion capture.

CLINICAL

Clinical outcome measures allowing the measurement of general posture include:

- Analysis of digital video by SiliconCOACH Pro version 6.0 program (2004)
- Matlab program 7.0 (Mathworks) software.

REFERENCES AND FURTHER READING

Carr J, Shepherd R: *Stroke rehabilitation guidelines for exercise and training to optimize motor skill*, Edinburgh, 2003, Butterworth-Heinemann.

Kandel ER, Schwartz JH, Jessell TM: *Principles of neural science*, ed 4, New York, 2000, McGraw-Hill Health professions Division.

Lennon S: Physiotherapy practice in stroke rehabilitation: a survey, *Disability and Rehabilitation* 259:455–461, 2003.

Marrone DF: Ultrastructural plasticity associated with hippocampal learning: a meta analysis, *Neurobiology of Learning and Memory* 873:361–371, 2007.

Mayston M: Handling and spasticity letter to the editor, *Physiotherapy* 86:559, 2000a.

Mayston M: Compensating for CNS dysfunction letter to the editor, *Physiotherapy* 86:612, 2000b.

SiliconCOACH: *SiliconCOACH coaching solutions for a digital age* [online]. New Zealand, 2004. www.siliconcoach.com (Accessed 1 September 2006).

Ungerleider LG, Doyon J, Karni A: Imaging brain plasticity during motor skill learning, *Neurobiology of Learning and Memory* 783:553–564, 2002.

21

Muscle tone

WHAT IS NORMAL MUSCLE TONE?

Muscle tone is often referred to as a state of readiness in a muscle at rest (resting tone) which provides us with a background level of tone from which we can function efficiently. It is defined by the resistance to passive movement, which is an expression of the stiffness of the muscle fibres (Brodal 2004). Normal tone should be high enough to keep you up against gravity but low enough to allow movement.

Caution

There is huge variation of normal within this definition. The ability to differentiate abnormal muscle tone can only come from an appreciation of this normal range and this requires the therapist to handle individuals with an intact nervous system.

When the limb of an individual with an intact central nervous system is moved passively the following characteristics are evident:

● The individual will 'follow' the movement (i.e. the muscles are active but allowing the movement to occur)
● The limb can be 'placed' at any point in the movement and will remain in its designated position.

In terms of muscle tone this requires the individual to reduce their muscle tone to a level that allows the limb to be moved freely (follow) but then to immediately recruit sufficient activity so that the limb remains in a position when released (placing).

Muscle tone is considered to depend physiologically on two factors:

● Non-neural
● Neural.

NON-NEURAL FACTORS

This is a consequence of the mechanical-elastic properties of the soft tissues (compliance or stiffness of soft tissue structures) and incorporates the thixotropic properties (viscosity) of the muscle and the muscle length. These factors contribute a significant component to the normal resting tone of a muscle which explains how we are able to stand still with only minimal corrective bursts of postural muscle activity (Simons and Mense 1998). These non-neural factors can be influenced by age, temperature and exercise.

NEURAL FACTORS

The neural factors relate to the degree of activation of the con-tractile apparatus of the muscle. Our muscles are constantly con-tracting or active and it is the nervous system that controls the appropriate level of this background activity. The level of muscle contraction is a result of the output from the alpha motor neuron (AMN) in the ventral horn of the spinal cord (S2.13) which innervates the muscle itself. The AMN output is dictated by the final outcome of competing inhibitory and excitatory synapses from various inputs related to both the peripheral and central nervous systems. These include:

- Muscle spindles (tonic component of the stretch reflex) (TSR) (S2.13)
- Golgi tendon organ (GTO) (S2.13)
- Somatosensory receptors in the body (skin, joints, connective tissue, muscles) (S3.23)
- Sensory systems such as visual, auditory, vestibular (S2.10)
- Limbic system related to our emotional state (S2.9)
- Other motor systems (S2.7)
- Interneurons within the spinal cord
- Various higher centres via the descending tracts (Reticular formation S2.10) (Nielsen et al. 2007).

It is the final assimilation of all these inputs at the level of the spinal cord which dictates the output from the alpha motor neuron and translates into the precise level of muscle tone.

WHAT IS ABNORMAL MUSCLE TONE?

Individuals who have a neurological lesions affecting the central nervous system (CNS) may lose the ability to control the level of muscle tone and may present with resting tone that is either too low (hypotonia) or too high (hypertonia) (Brodal 2004). It is also common to see both these characteristics present in an individual patient.

In CNS lesions, muscle weakness (S3.30) is evident in association with both hypotonia (reduced muscle tone) and hypertonia (increased muscle tone). The relationship between these concepts is complex but it appears likely that both altered tone states directly contribute to a reduction in force production (weakness) of the muscle. The pathophysiology which defines alterations in muscle tone will also lead to a dysfunction in the timing or pattern of motor unit recruitment or the number of units able to be recruited. This will lead to a presentation of muscle weakness during certain movements. It should also be noted that when altered tone exists over a prolonged period, the outcome may be disuse of the part, and further muscle weakness may occur as a consequence of sarcomere loss and reduction in cross-sectional area (S3.30).

In terms of assessment, a comparison of the conceptual definitions gives the therapist a simplified tool by which to differentiate muscle tone and weakness. Muscle tone is defined as the resistance to passive movement, representing the background level of tension or stiffness in a muscle (Moore and Kowalske 2000). Therefore it should be assessed in a muscle at rest. Muscle weakness on the other hand is defined as the inability to generate sufficient force to overcome the resistance of a task and therefore by definition should be assessed during movement activities.

HYPOTONIA

Definition

Hypotonia, or low tone, is a reduced level of muscle stiffness, providing little or no resistance when moved passively and which cannot be 'placed' on termination of the movement. The limb feels heavy when handled and tendon reflexes are reduced or absent. Patients with hypotonia will have difficulty staying up against gravity and when attempting to move present with areas of postural instability and ineffective muscle recruitment that makes movement effortful. An absence of muscle tone is referred to as flaccidity.

Pathophysiology of hypotonia

Hypotonia presents in many pathologies involving the central nervous system, e.g. multiple sclerosis, traumatic brain injury and cerebrovascular accident (CVA). Where an acute insult occurs, the nervous system may go into a state of neural shock (Kwakkel et al. 2003). The shock results in reduced neuronal conduction (S2.6) and a breakdown in communication within the nervous system. If the motor systems are affected, an insufficient number of alpha motor neurons can be recruited and hypotonia presents. Over time, as the nervous system recovers the neural shock subsides, neural transmission is resumed and muscle tone begins to return. However, there is no guarantee that it will return to normal.

If the patient still presents with hypotonia after a 4-week period, the presentation is sometimes termed 'prolonged muscular flaccidity' (Kwakkel et al. 2003). In CVA, the prognosis for the final outcome is poor if this state remains beyond 3 months (Formisano et al. 2005). The definitive cause of prolonged muscular flaccidity is unclear in the current literature. It has been hypothesized to result from a reduction in the levels of arousal and central drive leading to insufficient excitation at the alpha motor neuron. However, the cortical loops associated with the basal ganglia and cerebellum are also found to be severely affected in patients with prolonged muscular flaccidity (Pantano et al. 1995).

HYPERTONIA

Hypertonia, or high tone, is an increase in muscle stiffness with an increased resistance to passive movement. Patients often present with effortful movement that is often ineffective. Hypertonia is sub-divided into:

- Rigidity
- Hypertonia related to spasticity.

Rigidity defined

Traditionally, rigidity is defined as an increased resistance to passive movement which is constant throughout the range of movement. The resistance occurs throughout the full range of a passive movement and will be present in all muscles (including the face). The resistance is described as 'lead-pipe' (constant through range) or 'cogwheel' (resistance followed by a period of 'give') (Fung and Thompson 2002; Xia and Rymer 2004). As a result of rigidity affecting all muscle groups, patients often present with a lack of rotation, especially in the trunk (Wright et al. 2007). Recent studies have shown that rigidity is also velocity dependent (Mak et al. 2007; Xia et al. 2009). Voluntary movement is difficult both to initiate and arrest. Tendon reflexes are usually normal.

Pathophysiology of rigidity

Rigidity is one of the cardinal symptoms in Parkinson's disease (PD) but can be seen in any patient with a lesion of the basal ganglia. The presentation of increased resistance to passive movement in rigidity is a consequence of neural and non-neural factors.

Neural factors   The neural factors are a result of damage to the basal ganglia (S2.11) and particularly, the dopamine-producing cells of the substantia nigra (SN). The dopaminergic neurons of the SN project to the striatum and normally modulate the activity of both the direct and indirect pathways within the basal ganglia (S2.11), having the opposite effect on each. The direct pathway facilitates the initiation and selection of the correct voluntary movement programmes to achieve a task, while the indirect pathway helps to prevent any unwanted movement programmes. In PD, the loss of dopaminergic cells in the SN means that the ability to modulate motor programme selection is lost and there is inappropriate competition between the correct and incorrect movement programmes being sent to the cortex. At a muscular level, this presents as inappropriate co-contraction (Xia and Rymer 2004; Xia et al. 2009) attributed to inadequate reciprocal

Table 21.1 The positive and negative features of spasticity

Positive features	Negative features
Hyper-reflexia (S3.22)	Weakness (S3.30)
Hypertonia	Inability to fractionate
Gross movement patterns (S3.18)	Poor selective movement
Associated reactions (S3.18)	
Abnormal co-contraction	
Clonus (S3.18)	

inhibition (Meunier et al. 2000). Consequently, a hypokinetic movement disorder presents, or in simple terms a lack of movement.

Non-neural Altered muscle activity and joint movement leads to structural and functional changes in the musculoskeletal system. Muscles lose sarcomeres, becoming shorter, stiffer and more thixotropic and collagen production may be altered and disorganized. This structural change is considered to significantly contribute to the resistance to passive movement (Bhakta 2000; Chung et al. 2004; Vattanasilp et al. 2000).

Hypertonia (related to spasticity) defined

Hypertonia (related to spasticity) is notoriously difficult to understand for the novice therapist. This is primarily because in clinical practice the term 'spasticity' is often used interchangeably with hypertonia. This is misleading. Spasticity is defined as velocity- and length-dependent increase in the tonic stretch reflex with exaggerated tendon reflexes and is described as a range of positive and negative features (Table 21.1), one of which is hypertonia (Lance 1980; Platz et al. 2005; Burridge et al. 2005). Therefore, for clarity, this text will use the term 'hypertonia (related to spasticity)'. Hypertonia (related to spasticity) is defined as an increase in resistance to a passive movement that increases with the velocity of the movement and then fades away as the muscle is held in a constant stretch, when it is described as 'clasp knife'. The clinical presentation is a feeling of stiffness during part of or all of the range of movement and the patient's limb may be held in an abnormal posture. The pattern of hypertonia (related to spasticity) may be present in any muscle group, however common presentations have been linked with lesions of different levels of the brain:

Decorticate: a lesion at the level of the cerebral cortex (S2.7) or subcortical diencephalon (S2.9) the posture of hypertonia tends to be a flexor pattern of the upper limbs and an extensor pattern of the lower limbs (Magee 2002), the antigravity muscles.

Decerebrate: a lesion at the level of the brain stem (S2.10) the posture tends to be a predominance of extensor tone throughout (Kandel et al. 2000; Magee 2002).

Clinical observation seems to indicate that voluntary movement, increased effort and increased sensory stimulation may further increase hypertonia. However, evidence shows that in terms of reflex activity, this is not the case (Sharp and Brouwer 1997; Ada et al. 1998; Burne et al. 2005).

Pathophysiology of hypertonia (related to spasticity)

Hypertonia (related to spasticity) may be seen in patients with a lesion of the CNS. However, the nature of the pathology will dictate whether the onset is immediate (traumatic brain injury) or slowly evolving (CVA, multiple sclerosis, spinal cord injury) (Edwards 2002). The presentation of increased resistance to passive movement is related to a combination of neural and non-neural factors:

Neural factors   In terms of neural factors, hypertonia (related to spasticity) results from an increased excitability of the alpha motor neuron at the level of the spinal cord. This could occur as a consequence of (1) damage to inhibitory pathways (medullary or medial reticulospinal tract) or (2) increased activity of the excitatory pathways (pontine or lateral reticulospinal tract).

Interruption of the inhibitory pathways. Damage to the CNS, particularly the cortico-reticular pathway (Rathore 2002), results in reduced cortical drive to the inhibitory centre in the reticular formation (S2.10). The outcome is a release of the tonic stretch reflex (TSR) from higher centre inhibitory control (S2.13), which means that it becomes inappropriately responsive and muscle tone is increased. This is hypertonia. There is strong evidence linking spasticity with the release of the TSR in cerebral injury (Lin and Sabbahi 1999; Burne et al. 2005).

Increased activity of the excitatory pathways. Following damage to the nervous system, the surviving adjacent neurons undergo physiological changes which lead to structural adaptations (Nielsen et al. 2007). These adaptations are a result of neuroplastic processes which include denervation supersensitivity, collateral sprouting, unmasking and synaptic strengthening.

However, these processes do not necessarily lead to a positive functional outcome. In the case of spasticity, it is thought that increased sensitivity of the post-synaptic receptors on the remaining neurons and sprouting of adjacent dorsal root afferents can lead to an overall increase in excitatory inputs to the alpha motor neuron and hence hypertonia. This latter explanation of hypertonia could explain why hypertonia tends to develop over time (Sheean 2002).

Non-neural Altered muscle activity and joint movement leads to structural and functional changes in the musculoskeletal system. Muscles lose sarcomeres, becoming shorter, stiffer and more thixotropic and collagen production may be altered and disorganized. This structural change is considered to significantly contribute to the resistance to passive movement (Bhakta 2000; Chung et al. 2004; Vattanasilp et al. 2000).

In the literature, there remains uncertainty as to the relevant contributions of neural and non-neural factors. Electromyography studies show that the reflex-mediated increase in muscle tone reaches its maximum between 1 and 3 months post-lesion (Bhakta 2000; Teasell and Heitzner 1998), whereas others state that reflexic activity is only evident when a limb is moved quickly (Vattanasilp et al. 2000). However, after 3 months, the increased resistance to passive stretch is proposed to be primarily due to the intrinsic non-neural stiffness of the muscle (Bhakta 2000; Chung et al. 2004; Vattanasilp et al. 2000).

WHY DO I NEED TO ASSESS MUSCLE TONE?

It is important to assess muscle tone because of its potential effect on functional ability. Hypotonia appears to be a negative prognostic indicator in CVA and also prolongs the rehabilitation process (Formisano et al. 2005). A direct correlation between hypertonia and the level of disability has not been established (Sommerfeld et al. 2004) and little is known about hypertonia in a contracting muscle. In fact, some evidence implies that movement disorders observed in patients who present with hypertonia are the result of weakness in the agonist muscle rather than hypertonia in the antagonist. It is therefore unclear how, or if, hypertonia contributes directly to the movement disorders itself. However, a detrimental effect on function has been associated with the secondary side-effects of hypertonia, which include pain (Pizzi 2005), contracture (Watkins et al. 2002; Pizzi 2005), limitation of range of movement (Lin and Sabbahi 1999) and muscle weakness (Maruishi et al. 2001).

HOW DO I ASSESS MUSCLE TONE?

OBSERVATION

Patient

The therapist may start their assessment of muscle tone in any posture but will need to assess in various postures to gain a true insight into the patient's deficit.

Therapist

1. The therapist should observe:
   a. Muscle bulk
   b. Skin creases
   c. Movement patterns
2. Where relevant comparing both sides to evaluate.

Caution

It is often recommended during assessment of CVA to compare the affected side with the non-affected side. However, caution is advised because of motor/sensory tracts which remain ipsilateral (i.e. do not decussate). This means that both sides may be affected by the lesion.

Are left and right sides similar in terms of muscle bulk? Increased muscle bulk may be indicative of hypertonia, where hypertrophy has occurred. Decreased muscle bulk may signify hypotonia. These signs are not definitive because other factors can produce differences in bulk between sides (e.g. handedness and level, type and frequency of functional activities).

Are there asymmetrical excessive skin creases present (Fig. 21.1)? These may indicate that the underlying muscle is underactive due to hypotonia.

Does the patient present with any abnormal patterns of movement (S3.18)? Signs of hypotonia relate to postural instability, the inability to stabilize body segments against the effects of gravity. Therapists often evaluate active movement looking for gross patterns of movement, increased effort and associated reactions as signs of spasticity, however although hypertonia is often associated with these signs, there is no evidence to suggest a

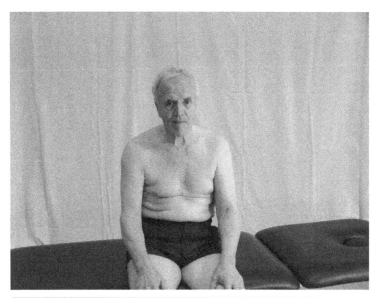

Figure 21.1 Skin creases in sitting.

direct link (Ada and O'Dwyer 2001; Bhakta et al. 2001). The novice therapist should therefore be clear about what is being evaluated and why.

PALPATION

Therapist

1. Palpate the muscles
2. When relevant, compare with the other side.

How does the muscle tension feel? Excessive tension could relate to hypertonia and reduced tension linked to hypotonia. However, this is weak evidence of its existence.

PASSIVE MOVEMENTS

Therapist

This tool assesses the resistance to passive movement and therefore adheres closely to the definition of altered muscle tone. The therapist is evaluating the overall outcome of both the neural and non-neural components of muscle tone. The test should be carried out with the muscle at rest, therefore ensure that the patient is comfortable and supported.

Caution
Some patients may find it very difficult to fully relax. The consequent tension in the muscles is not hypertonia.

Limb testing

1. Support the full weight of the limb to be tested (Figs 21.2, 21.3).

 Caution
All passive movement should be carried out slowly and carefully at first. If the muscle tone is low there is a risk of causing damage to the soft tissue structures surrounding the joint.

2. Move the limb slowly through its full range of motion.
3. Re-evaluate that the movement is passive (no effort on the part of the patient).
4. The therapist may need to repeat the movement, however this should be kept to a minimum as movement may influence the non-neural component in hypertonic muscles.
5. If hypertonia is suspected an increase in the speed of the passive movement may help in confirming the diagnosis. This specifically tests the reflex component of muscle stiffness. The velocity-dependent hypertonic muscle then offers greater resistance.
6. Repeat the passive movements in all directions of movement and for all joints, including both upper and lower limb. For example, at the shoulder, assess medial/lateral rotation, abduction/adduction and flexion/extension.

 Caution
This technique is potentially a high-risk manual handling task. Please manage the risk as appropriate.

Trunk testing   This involves performing a passive movement to the patient's trunk.

1. This can be achieved with the patient in sitting (Fig. 21.4) but equally well in side lying (Fig. 21.5).
2. The trunk/thorax should be moved in all directions in relation to the pelvis in order to assess the resistance in the trunk muscles.

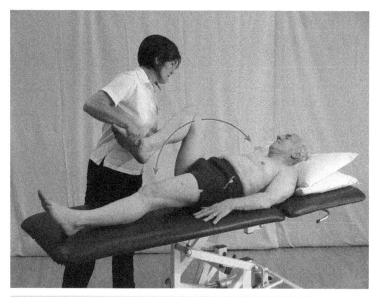

Figure 21.2 Assessing muscle tone (lower limbs).

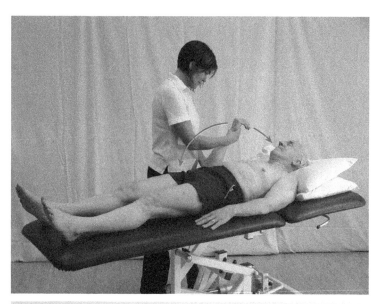

Figure 21.3 Assessing muscle tone (upper limbs).

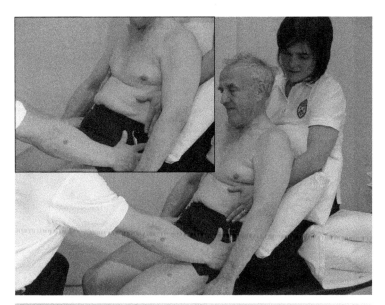

Figure 21.4 Assessing muscle tone (trunk) in sitting.

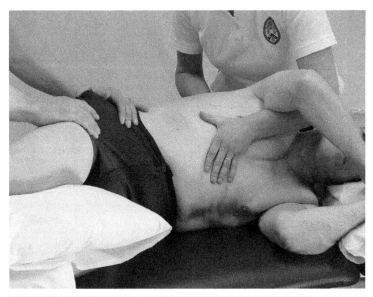

Figure 21.5 Assessing muscle tone (trunk) in side lying.

3. In order to carry this out effectively, one segment (pelvis) may need to be stabilized while the other (trunk) is moved. This will require two therapists.

Is there any resistance to the passive movement? Yes, indicates hypertonia. No, indicates normal tone or hypotonia.

At what point in the movement is the resistance felt? Hypertonia associated with spasticity can occur in part of the movement range or throughout range, whereas that associated with rigidity occurs throughout the full range.

Are there any defining characteristics to the resistance offered? Clasp knife (related to spasticity) or cog wheel/lead pipe related to rigidity. Hypertonia in all muscle groups is indicative of rigidity, whereas a presentation confined to particular muscle groups is likely to be hypertonia (related to spasticity).

Does the resistance increase if the speed of the passive movement is increased? This velocity-dependent change indicates hypertonia, but it could be spasticity or rigidity.

Does the limb feel heavy and provide little or no resistance to the movement? This is hypotonia.

REFLEX TESTING

Therapist

Reflex testing (S3.22) is carried out to evaluate or confirm the integrity of the reflex pathway and the reflexic properties of the muscle. This may tell us in part about the neural component of muscle tone but it does not tell us about the overall stiffness of a muscle. Therefore it is an inappropriate tool to use for testing muscle tone in isolation. In terms of hypo-reflexia, the peripheral or central nervous system could be implicated. A hyper-reflexic muscle may confirm the involvement spasticity, however caution is advised when directly relating this finding to hypertonia as the evidence indicates that there is a low correlation between the existence of hypertonia and increased tendon jerk reflexes (S2.22) (Teasell and Heitzner 1998).

RECORDING

When recording findings, the therapist may use a body chart (Fig. 21.6) or a text description (Table 21.2).

Example

See Figure 21.6 and Table 21.2.

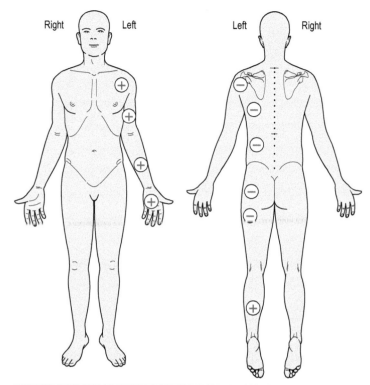

Figure 21.6 Example of a body chart recording (muscle tone).

Table 21.2 Example of a text description recording (muscle tone)
Patient in sitting:
Left side of trunk shows no resistance to movement in any direction.
Left UL: Subluxation of the glenohumeral joint. No resistance to passive movements of the shoulder complex. Increased resistance through middle range of elbow extension and wrist and finger extension.
Right UL: Normal tone.
Left LL: No resistance to movements of the hip/pelvis and increased resistance through range of dorsiflexion.
Right LL: Normal tone.

ANALYSIS

The identification of severe hypotonia or hypertonia is often uncomplicated. However, in moderate and mild severity, diagnosis is more difficult. The differential diagnosis of rigidity and spasticity will primarily be based upon the area of brain damaged. However, based on the pathophysiology of altered muscle tone which identifies both neural and non-neural components, the therapist should use a combination of assessment tools before coming to a conclusion. The therapist should also assess the patient for any other (treatable) factors which may be influencing muscle tone, such as, pain (musculoskeletal or systemic), soft tissue adaptation (from poor seating), medication or emotional stress. These should be alleviated as a priority.

Analysis of the example shown in Figure 21.6 and Table 21.2 leads to the hypothesis that hypotonia exists through the left trunk, shoulder and hip girdles, with hypertonia evident in the flexor muscles of the left elbow, wrist and hand and in the extensor muscles of the left ankle.

OUTCOME MEASURES

RESEARCH
- Electromyography (EMG)
- H reflex.

CLINICAL
As altered muscle tone is defined by description of its stiffness, a measurement of resistance to passive movement is most accurate.

- Modified Ashworth Scale
- Tardieu Scale
- Modified Tardieu Scale.

REFERENCES AND FURTHER READING
Ada L, O'Dwyer N: Do associated reactions in the upper limb after stroke contribute to contracture? *Clinical Rehabilitation* 15:186–194, 2001.
Ada L, Vattanasilp W, O'Dwyer N, et al: Does spasticity contribute to walking dysfunction after stroke? *Journal of Neurology Neurosurgery and Psychiatry* 64:628–635, 1998.
Bhakta BB: Management of spasticity in stroke, *British Medical Bulletin* 56:476–485, 2000.

Bhakta BB, Cozens JA, Chamberlain MA, et al: Quantifying associated reactions in the paretic arm in stroke and their relationship to spasticity, *Clinical Rehabilitation* 15:195–206, 2001.

Brodal P: *The central nervous system: structure and function*, ed 3, Oxford, 2004, Oxford University Press.

Burne JA, Carleton VL, O'Dwyer NJ: The spasticity paradox: movement disorder or disorder of resting limbs? *Journal of Neurology Neurosurgery and Psychiatry* 76:47–54, 2005.

Burridge JH, Wood DE, Hermens HJ, et al: Theoretical and methodological considerations in the measurement of spasticity, *Disability and Rehabilitation* 271/2:69–80, 2005.

Chung SG, van Rey E, Bai Z, et al: Biomechanic changes in passive properties of hemiplegic ankles with spastic hypertonia, *Archives of Physical Medicine and Rehabilitation* 85:1638–1646, 2004.

Corden DM, Lippold OC, Buchanan K, et al: Long-latency component of the stretch reflex in human muscle is not mediated by intramuscular stretch receptors, *Journal of Neurophysiology* 84:184–188, 2000.

Edwards S: *Neurological physiotherapy*, Edinburgh, 2002, Churchill Livingstone.

Formisano R, Pantano P, Buzzi MG, et al: Late motor recovery is influenced by muscle tone changes after stroke, *Archives of Physical Medicine and Rehabilitation* 86:308–311, 2005.

Fung VS, Thompson PD: Rigidity and spasticity. In: Jankovic JJ, Tolosa E, editors. *Parkinson's disease and movement disorders*, ed 4, Philadelphia, 2002, Lippincott Williams and Wilkins, pp 473–482.

Kandel ER, Schwartz JH, Jessell TM: *Principles of neural science*, ed 4, New York, 2000, McGraw-Hill.

Kwakkel G, Kollen BJ, van der Grond J, et al: Probability of regaining dexterity in the flaccid upper limb: impact of severity of paresis and time since onset in acute stroke, *Stroke* 34:2181–2186, 2003.

Lance JW: Spasticity: disordered motor control. In: Feldman RG, Young RR, Koella WP, editors. *Spasticity: disordered motor control*, Chicago, 1980, Year Book Medical, pp 485–494.

Lin F-M, Sabbahi M: Correlation of spasticity with hyperactive stretch reflexes and motor dysfunction in hemiplegia, *Archives of Physical Medicine and Rehabilitation* 80:526–530, 1999.

Magee DJ: *Orthopaedic physical assessment*, ed 4, Canada, 2002, Elsevier Sciences.

Mak MK, Wong EC, Hui-Chan CW: Quantitative measurement of trunk rigidity in parkinsonian patients, *Journal of Neurology* 254:202–209, 2007.

Maruishi M, Mano Y, Sasaki T, et al: Cerebral palsy in adults: independent effects of muscle strength and muscle tone, *Archives of Physical Medicine and Rehabilitation* 82:637–641, 2001.

Meunier S, Pol S, Houeto JL, et al: Abnormal reciprocal inhibition between antagonist muscles in Parkinson's disease, *Brain* 123:1017–1026, 2000.

Moore DP, Kowalske KJ: Neuromuscular rehabilitation and electrodiagnosis of myopathy, *Archives of Physical Medicine and Rehabilitation* 81:S-32–S-35, 2000.

Nielsen JB, Crone C, Hultborn H: The spinal pathophysiology of spasticity – from a basic science point of view, *Acta Physiologica* 1892:171–18010, 2007.

Pantano P, Formisano R, Ricci M, et al: Prolonged muscular flaccidity after stroke: morphological and functional brain alterations, *Brain* 118:1329–1338, 1995.

Platz T, Eickhof C, Nuyens G, et al: Clinical scales for the assessment of spasticity associated phenomena and function: a systematic review of the literature, *Disability and Rehabilitation* 271/2: 7–18, 2005.

Pizzi A, Carlucci G, Falsini C, et al: Evaluation of upper-limb spasticity after stroke: a clinical and neurophysiologic study, *Archives of Physical Medicine and Rehabilitation* 86:410–415, 2005.

Rathore SS, Hinn AR, Cooper LS, et al: Characterization of incident stroke signs and symptoms: findings from the Atherosclerosis Risk in Communities Study, *Stroke* 33:2718–2721, 2002.

Sharp SA, Brouwer BJ: Isokinetic strength training of the hemiparetic knee: effects on function and spasticity, *Archives of Physical Medicine and Rehabilitation* 78:1231–1236, 1997.

Sheean G: The pathophysiology of spasticity, *European Journal of Neurology* 9:3–9, 2002.

Simons DG, Mense S: Understanding and measurement of muscle tone as related to clinical muscle pain, *Pain* 75:1–17, 1998.

Sommerfeld DK, EekE U-B, Svensson A-K, et al: Spasticity after stroke: its occurrence and association with motor impairments and activity limitations, *Stroke* 35:134–140, 2004.

Teasell RW, Heitzner JD: The painful hemiplegic shoulder, *Physical Medicine and Rehabilitation: State of the Art* 12:489–500, 1998.

Vattanasilp W, Ada L, Crosbie J: Contribution of thixotropy spasticity and contracture to ankle stiffness after stroke, *Journal of Neurology Neurosurgery and Psychiatry* 69:34–39, 2000.

Watkins C, Leathley M, Gregson J, et al: Prevalence of spasticity post stroke, *Clinical Rehabilitation* 165:515–522, 2002.

Woollacott AJ, Burne JA: The tonic stretch reflex and spastic hypertonia after spinal cord injury, *Experimental Brain Research* 1742:386–396, 2006.

Wright WG, Gurfinkel VS, Nutt J, et al: Axial hypertonicity in Parkinson's disease: direct measurements of trunk and hip torque, *Experimental Neurology* 208:38–46, 2007.

Xia R, Rymer WZ: Reflex reciprocal facilitation of antagonist muscles in spinal cord injury, *Spinal Cord* 43:14–21, 2004.

Xia R, Sun S, Threlkeld J: Analysis of interactive effect of stretch reflex and shortening reaction on rigidity in Parkinson's disease, *Clinical Neurophysiology* 120:1400–1407, 2009.

Reflexes

WHAT IS REFLEX TESTING?

Reflex testing, commonly referred to as a tendon jerk, involves evaluating the response of the phasic component of the stretch reflex pathway (S2.13). The test is referred to as a tendon reflex because a sharp stretch applied to the tendon by the therapist produces a corresponding stretch in most or all of the stretch receptors (muscle spindles) within the muscle itself. The result is temporal summation of the excitatory action potentials (S2.6) at the alpha motor neuron, which leads to a muscle contraction.

WHY DO I NEED TO ASSESS REFLEXES?

Assessing reflexes can give the therapist important information related to:

NERVE INTEGRITY

By testing the reflex arc, the therapist is assessing the integrity of the neural pathway from the spinal cord to the muscle and vice versa. This is crucial information in conditions affecting the lower motor neuron pathway or peripheral nervous system, such as spinal cord injury, motor neuron disease or Guillain–Barré syndrome. An absent response indicates a complete lesion somewhere along the neural pathway or in the muscle itself.

REFLEXIC PROPERTIES OF THE MUSCLE

Having established that the neural pathway is intact, the *muscle response* can also provide useful information to the therapist.

Hyper-reflexia

A brisk response to testing is termed an exaggerated reflex or hyper-reflexia and is one of the positive signs of spasticity (S3.21). Hyper-reflexia is considered to be a consequence of reduced descending inhibition from the cerebral cortex and in particular is associated with damage to the cortico-reticulospinal pathway (Rathore et al. 2002). The presentation of hyper-reflexia therefore implies a lesion of the central nervous system (CNS) and is cause for concern in disorders where CNS damage would not be initially suspected.

Hypo-reflexia

A diminished response to testing is termed hypo-reflexia and may be observed in pathologies affecting either the central or peripheral nervous system. More specifically it can relate to a lesion of one or more components of the reflex arc, the modulating descending systems or the muscle itself (Kandel et al. 2000).

 Caution

Caution is advised when analysing the reflexic properties of muscle as this property is influenced by many other factors such as tension and anxiety.

 HOW DO I ASSESS REFLEXES?

TENDON JERK

Patient

The patient should be comfortable and relaxed so that the testing can be completed with the muscle in a resting state. The position will therefore alter depending upon the muscle being tested.

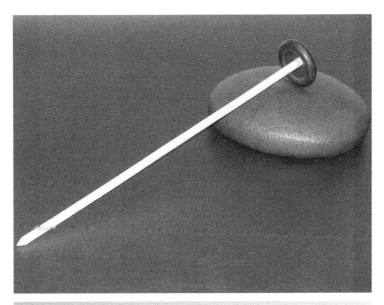

Figure 22.1 The reflex hammer.

Therapist

1. Reflexes are assessed using a reflex hammer (Fig. 22.1).
2. Palpate the tendon to be tested to establish the point of contact for the reflex hammer.
3. The hammer is held loosely with the handle uppermost allowing momentum to swing the hammer freely.
4. The head of the hammer is then used gently to apply a stretch to the tendon of the relevant muscle.

Biceps (C5, C6) (Fig. 22.2)
    a. The patient's arm should be flexed at the elbow with the palm down
    b. Place a thumb or finger firmly on the biceps tendon
    c. Strike your finger with the reflex hammer
    d. Note any elbow flexion.

Triceps (C6, C7) (Fig. 22.3)
    a. Support the upper arm in a position of 90° abduction. Then let the patient's forearm hang free
    b. Strike the triceps tendon above the elbow with the hammer
    c. Note any elbow extension.

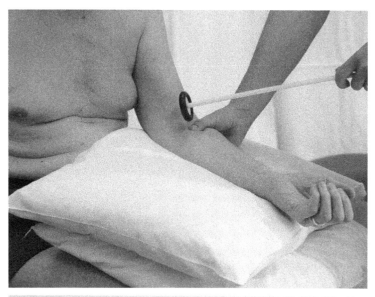

Figure 22.2 Tendon jerk testing for biceps.

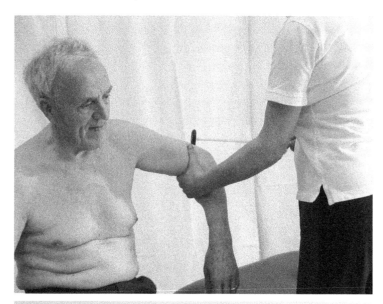

Figure 22.3 Tendon jerk testing for triceps.

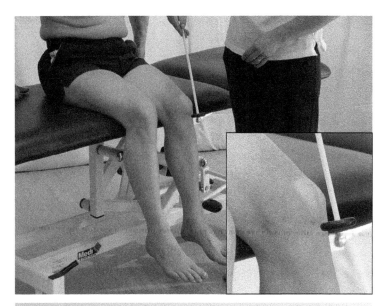

Figure 22.4 Tendon jerk testing for quadriceps femoris.

Quadriceps (L2, L3, L5) (Fig. 22.4)
    a. Have the patient sit or lie down with the knee relaxed and flexed
    b. Strike the patellar tendon just below the patella
    c. Note any knee extension.

Plantar flexors (S1, S2) (Fig. 22.5)
    a. Position the patient in long sitting or prone. Dorsiflex the foot at the ankle
    b. Strike the Achilles tendon
    c. Note any plantar flexion at the ankle.

★ Caution
Reflex response depends on the force of your stimulus. Use no more force than you need to provoke a definite response.

5. The response may be graded as follows:
    – or 0 absent
    – or 1 diminished
    + or 2 normal/average
    ++ or 3 brisk
    +++ or 4 exaggerated.

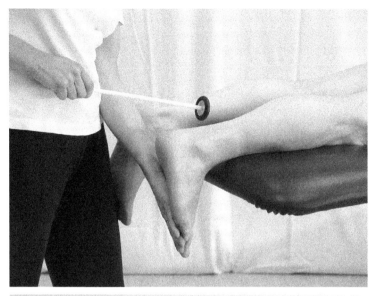

Figure 22.5 Tendon jerk testing for plantar flexors.

Does the muscle being tested respond at all? Yes, the neural pathway and muscle are intact for the spinal root levels indicated. For example, an appropriate response from biceps indicates that levels $C_{5,6}$ are intact. If there is no response, then a lesion involving the neural pathway at the same levels should be suspected.

How does the muscle respond? A response greater than 2 indicates hyper-reflexia and therefore it may be wise to look for other signs of spasticity (e.g. hypertonia). A diminished response indicates hypo-reflexia.

PLANTAR RESPONSE (BABINSKI SIGN) (FIG. 22.6)

Patient
The patient should be in supine or long sitting and be well supported so that the testing can be completed with the muscles of the lower limb in a resting state.

Therapist
1. Using the end of a reflex hammer
2. Draw the end upwards along the lateral border of the foot
3. At the base of the 5th toe move medially across the ball of the foot (Fig. 22.6)

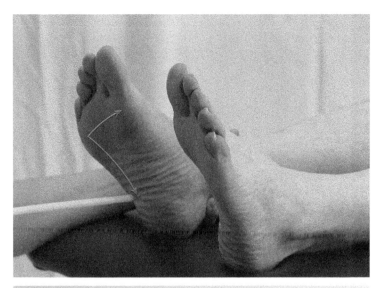

Figure 22.6 Testing for the Babinski sign.

4. This is performed in a continuous movement and at a fairly quick speed
5. Note the movement of the toes
6. A normal response is flexion (withdrawal). Extension of the big toe with fanning of the other toes is abnormal. This is referred to as a positive Babinski sign and is indicative of a lesion of the central nervous system.

RECORDING

Recording by the therapist usually consists of a simple list comprising the muscle tested and the response gained. For example:

- Biceps – Brisk or ++ or 3
- Quads – Diminished or – or 1
- Babinski – Negative.

ANALYSIS

It is important to remember that the findings from reflex testing need to be considered alongside other assessment findings. For example, in pathologies affecting the peripheral nervous system analysis should be in conjunction with results from the assessments of myotomes (S3.31) and dermatomes (S3.24). In pathologies affecting the central nervous system analysis may be in conjunction with findings related to the assessment of muscle tone (S3.21).

OUTCOME MEASURE

RESEARCH
- H reflex.

CLINICAL
- Tendon jerk testing
- Babinski sign.

REFERENCES AND FURTHER READING

Kandel ER, Schwartz JH, Jessell TM: *Principles of neural science*, ed 4, New York, 2000, McGraw-Hill.

Petty NJ: *Neuromusculoskeletal examination and assessment: a handbook for therapists*, Edinburgh, 2006, Churchill Livingstone.

Rathore SS, Hinn AR, Cooper LS, et al: Characterization of incident stroke signs and symptoms: findings from the Atherosclerosis Risk in Communities Study, *Stroke* 33:2718–2721, 2002.

Sensation

WHAT IS SENSATION?

Sensation is complex, consisting of several modalities, namely the four special senses (vision, hearing, smell and taste) and our somatosensory senses (tactile (light touch and pressure), proprioception, temperature and nociception/pain). Our sensory experience is a construct of the brain, which perceives and attaches meaning to these sensory modalities. Although all these modalities are relevant to function and our quality of life, only the somatosensory senses are covered in this section. Somatosensory information allows us to experience the environment, warns us of potential danger and is fundamental in maintaining arousal and the control of movement.

SENSORY RECEPTORS

The somatosensory system reacts to diverse stimuli from different sensory receptors, thermoreceptors (temperature), mechanoreceptors (physical distortion) and chemoreceptors (chemicals). Each sensory modality has a unique sensory receptor which is activated when a specific stimulus, within its receptive field, reaches a threshold intensity. This receptive field may be altered as a result of pathology when it can contribute to the experience of pain (S3.29) and abnormal sensation. The density of receptors is relevant to the ability to locate a stimulus (awareness) and to distinguish between two stimuli (discrimination).

The duration of a sensory experience is related to a further characteristic of the sensory receptor termed 'adaptation'. A rapidly adapting receptor responds to change and is therefore activated at the onset and termination of the stimulus only. A slowly adapting receptor responds continuously to a persistent stimulus. This should be borne in mind when assessing particular modalities. Figure 23.1 shows the main somatosensory receptors and Table 23.1 identifies the functional characteristics of these receptors.

SENSORY PATHWAY

This afferent information from sensory receptors in the periphery is conducted along afferent neurons to the spinal cord (S2.13) and transmitted via the ascending tracts (S2.15) to the thalamus (S2.9), brain stem (S2.10) and higher centres (S2.7). Sensory input is systematically mapped on the contralateral primary somatosensory cortex (parietal lobe), then processed and integrated with other relevant information by the somatosensory association area (parietal lobe), basal ganglia (S2.11) and cerebellum (S2.12) before being acted upon.

 Clinical hints and tips

Functionally relevant information is often transmitted in the same anatomical ascending tract (S2.15) but in separate parallel pathways. For example, when holding an object, the information related to texture (light touch) and shape (proprioception) are both conveyed in the dorsal columns. This overlap in function may be important clinically as following a lesion, the adjacent preserved tracts may be able to assist in the lost function.

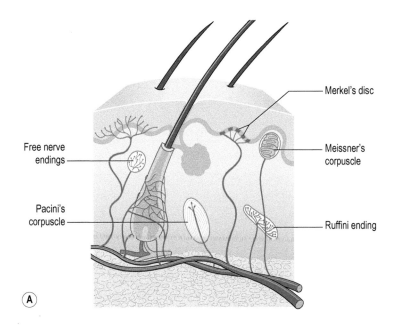

Merkel's disc

Free nerve endings

Meissner's corpuscle

Pacini's corpuscle

Ruffini ending

(A)

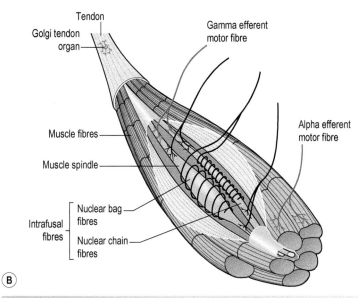

Tendon

Golgi tendon organ

Gamma efferent motor fibre

Muscle fibres

Alpha efferent motor fibre

Muscle spindle

Intrafusal fibres

Nuclear bag fibres

Nuclear chain fibres

(B)

Figure 23.1 Sensory receptors of the skin and muscle.

Table 23.1 Summary of the characteristics of somatosensory receptors

Sensory receptor	Function	Rapid adapting (RA)/Slow adapting (SA)	Receptive field
Ruffini ending (subcutaneous)	Stretch of skin and monitors skin slippage during functional grip	SA	Large
Meissner's corpuscles (superficial)	Light touch of skin. Highly sensitive to vibration	RA	Small
Pacinian corpuscles (subcutaneous)	Pressure in skin	RA	Large
Merkel's disc (superficial)	Sustained light touch and pressure in skin	SA	Small

SENSORY MODALITIES

Table 23.2 shows a summary of the functional anatomy related to the modalities described below.

Tactile

In terms of touch a hierarchy of sensory function was proposed by Fess (1990). The lowest level is the ability to identify a single stimulus (awareness). The hierarchy proceeds with the ability to distinguish between two stimuli (discrimination), the ability to differentiate different characteristics or strength of one stimulus (quantification) and the highest level is the ability to recognize objects by touch alone (recognition). This hierarchy suggests that if the higher levels are intact, the lower levels do not need to be assessed.

Light touch The sensation of light touch allows us to be aware of tactile stimuli, including situations as innocuous as the clothes we wear, but also has a role in warning us of impending damage. Following a neurological lesion, a patient may become hypersensitive to touch, when even clothes may initiate a sensory experience and an inappropriate motor response. This altered sensation may also be perceived as pain, paraesthesia or dysaesthesia (S3.29). In

Table 23.2 Summary of sensory modalities and their relevant functional anatomy

Modality	Sub-modality	Sensory receptor	Nerve fibre	Ascending tract
Tactile	Light touch	Meissner's corpuscle and Merkel's discs	A beta	Dorsal columns
	Deep touch (pressure)	Pacinian corpuscles	A beta	Dorsal columns
Proprioception	Position sense	Muscle spindle (primary and secondary endings): Ruffini endings: *minor role for joint receptors.*	A beta	Dorsal columns. Spinocerebellar
	Movement sense	Muscle spindle (primary ending) Ruffini endings in skin	A beta	
	Force	Muscle spindle (primary and secondary endings)	A beta and A gamma	
Nociception	Pain	Free nerve endings:		Spinothalamic
	Temperature	Mechanical and thermal (sharp pain)	A delta	Spinoreticular
	Tactile (crude)	Mechanical, thermal (>45°) and chemical (slow burning pain)	C fibre	Spinotectal

a scenario where a patient becomes hyposensitive to light touch, the lack of awareness of limbs particularly, may result in soft tissue injury.

Pressure/deep touch   As for light touch, our sense of pressure is important in avoiding tissue damage, performing functional activities such as grip and weight bearing activities but is also likely to contribute to proprioception.

Two-point discrimination   This is the ability to identify two objects in contact with the skin as two distinct points, rather than one. Lesions of the sensory cortex may result in difficulty discriminating two points within the normal distances (finger tips 2–4 mm; palm 8–15 mm; back 30–40 mm) and this increased two-point discrimination has been found to be a poor prognostic indicator for recovery in cerebrovascular accident (CVA).

Graphesthesia   This is the ability to recognize writing on the skin purely through the medium of touch. This ability requires integration by the higher centres with other sensory information and in relation to past experience (memory).

Clinical hints and tips
Tactile discrimination requires an intact somatosensory system and the ability to process and integrate the input with other information/systems. Therefore, a deficit of discriminatory skill could implicate various regions of the central nervous system.

Nociception

Pain (S3.29)   Pain serves to notify the nervous system about tissue damage that has occurred. Although pain can be elicited without tissue damage (neurogenic pain) (S3.29), nociceptive pain will remain the focus here. The sensory receptors sensitive to nociceptive stimuli are free nerve endings, however not all noxious stimuli is perceived as pain because the response to a stimuli is highly subjective. The free nerve endings are much less specialized than other receptors and may respond to mechanical, thermal or chemical stimuli.

Temperature

Our sense of skin temperature is protective in avoiding tissue damage and is anatomically and functionally closely related to pain.

Proprioception

Our sense of proprioception is complex and results from integration of information from several sources, visual (S2.10, S3.27), vestibular (S2.10) and somatosensory systems. In this text, proprioception is defined as consisting of three sub-modalities (Riemann and Lephart 2002a,b); the ability to sense:

- Position sense (body parts and their relationship to each other)
- Movement sense (sometimes referred to as kinaesthesia)
- Force.

Proprioception also governs the ability to recognize an object using the sense of touch through manipulation (stereognosis). This sense is mediated via the dorsal columns, however the ability to recognize any object requires integration by the higher centres with other sensory information and in relation to past experience (memory).

Historically, joint receptors have been considered to have an important role in proprioception, however recent studies have shown that this is not the case in most joints (Proske and Gandevia 2009). In fact, the major sensory receptors involved in position and movement sense are muscle spindles and stretch receptors in the skin (Ruffini endings). The skin receptors have a greater role in circumstances where the controlling muscle is distant to the joint being moved (e.g. fingers) (Collins et al. 2005) and in the case of two joint muscles (Sturnieks et al. 2007). Ruffini endings have been found to be accurate within 2° in relation to change of joint angle in the fingers and deficits contribute to altered timing and force of grip in stroke (Blennerhassett et al. 2007).

WHY DO I NEED TO ASSESS SENSATION?

A lesion of the somatosensory system is likely to impact greatly on the neurologically impaired patient. For example:

- Inability to interact with the environment
- Risk of soft tissue damage
- Inability to produce skilled movement (Campbell 2000)
- Significant reduction in functional ability (Fang et al. 2003, Tyson et al. 2008) and quality of life (Forsaa et al. 2008)
- Production of central neuropathic pain (S3.29) (Widerstrom-Noga et al. 2002).

The incidence of sensory deficit is also high in this patient population. In Parkinson's disease (PD), there is a growing body of evidence that suggests that non-motor symptoms such as abnormal sensation may actually precede the motor deficits by which it is presently diagnosed. Between 50% and 100% of people with PD have sensory deficits (Rahman et al. 2008) with a decrease in two-point discrimination and proprioception highlighted (Zia et al. 2000). This is attributed to an impairment of sensorimotor processing by the basal ganglia (S2.11) (Juri et al. 2009).

In CVA and multiple sclerosis (MS) the lesion may directly involve the somatosensory system or the processing centres and therefore may result in a dysfunction of any of the somatosensory modalities. The incidence is up to 60% in CVA (Schabrun and Hillier 2009) with tactile deficits most common and considered a poor prognostic indicator for recovery (Tyson et al. 2008).

HOW DO I ASSESS SENSATION?

The primary modalities that should be part of a neurological assessment include light touch, deep touch/pressure, temperature, pain and proprioception (Cassiopeia and Okun 2002). In order to save time, clinicians may opt to assess pain *or* temperature (anterior spinothalamic tract), light touch *or* deep touch (dorsal columns) and proprioception.

The patient may report that they are aware of an area of numbness or altered sensation during the subjective assessment. This can then be explored during the objective assessment. Although the following procedures are subjective in nature, they do reflect current clinical practice.

TACTILE – LIGHT TOUCH

Patient
Position the patient in a comfortable supported position suitably undressed to access as much skin as possible, while maintaining dignity.

Therapist
1. Decide on the distribution of testing
   - *Peripheral nervous system (PNS) lesion* testing dermatomes (S3.24) (Fig. 23.2) or peripheral nerve distribution (Fig. 23.3) will give the therapist the most useful information.

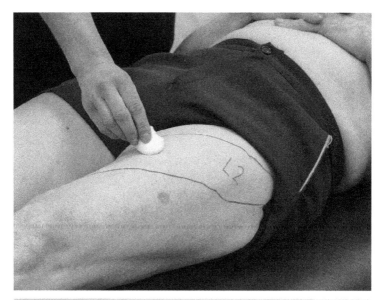

Figure 23.2 Testing a dermatome for light touch.

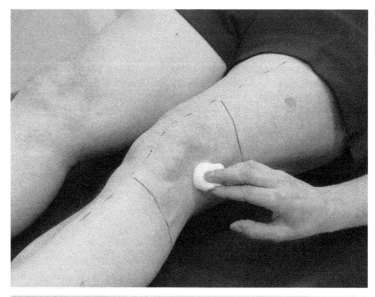

Figure 23.3 Testing a peripheral nerve for light touch.

- *Central nervous system (CNS) lesion.* Any sensory loss will be due to damage affecting the sensory homunculus and therefore is likely to correlate to body segments. Therefore, testing the distribution of peripheral nerves or dermatomes is neither necessary nor relevant. Testing the area of skin related to different aspects (medial, lateral, anterior, posterior) of particular body segments is more accurate in terms of the pathophysiology and provides clear landmarks by which the patient can report localization of the stimuli. For example, front of the elbow (Fig. 23.4), back of the wrist, inside of the knee and outside of the ankle.

2. Explain and demonstrate the procedure to the patient with their eyes open.
3. Test an area of skin considered to be normal to ensure the patient understands what is expected.
4. Ask the patient to close their eyes.
5. Using a cotton wool ball, touch the area of skin being assessed (Figs 23.2–23.4). A brief dab will activate the rapid adapting Meissner's corpuscles, whereas a sustained application of the cotton wool will stimulate the slow adapting Merkel's disc.
6. Compare the same area of skin on the other side.

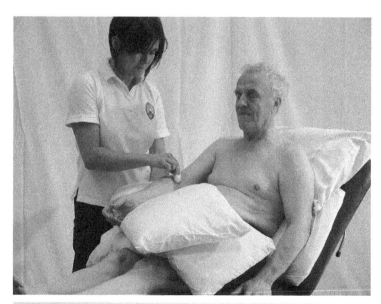

Figure 23.4 Testing segmental distribution for light touch.

Caution
Try not to drag the cotton wool as this will evoke sensory receptors in the hair follicles and provide the patient with additional sensory information. Therefore the therapist will not gain a true reflection of light touch.

Clinical hints and tips
Sensory testing should be carried out bilaterally. However, in pathologies where both sides may be affected, the therapist should compare to expected normative levels.

7. The therapist should encourage the patient not to try and guess if they are not sure about accuracy. With this in mind the therapist is advised to randomize the testing points in terms of the body segment tested and the timing of the test.
8. Ask the patient to respond as follows:
   Say 'yes' every time you feel me touch you. This evaluates sensory awareness. A correct 'yes' response, indicates that the sensory pathway itself is intact. If there is no response, the area is likely to be anaesthetic (lacks sensation). This could indicate dysfunction of either the peripheral or central nervous systems.

Clinical hints and tips
For patients with verbal communication deficits, a strategy such as blinking or raising a finger may be substituted. If possible the patient could also point to establish the ability to localize the sensation.

9. Further questioning at the same test point may allow the therapist to establish more detail which will assist clinical reasoning later:
   Does it feel normal? No, it feels strange. This could be peripheral or central neuropathic pain and needs further exploration (S3.29).
   Does it feel the same as the other side? No. What is different? Which side feels normal? This could indicate an ipsilateral peripheral nervous system lesion or a contralateral central nervous system lesion.
   Tell me where I am touching you This tests the ability to localize (identify the location of) the sensation. Inability to

localize the stimuli implicates a lesion of the primary somatosensory cortex (parietal lobe).

10. Record any loss or change in normal sensation.

11. To ensure nothing is missed, the procedure should be
repeated to include the whole body (limbs and trunk) bilaterally. However, a recent study by Busse and Tyson (2009)
recommended that in CVA, if *one* site on a limb was assessed
as either completely absent or intact, no further testing of
that limb was required. However, if the segment was assessed
as partially impaired, the whole limb should be tested.

12. The therapist should then go on to test:
    - Two-point discrimination (discrimination)
    - Different textures (quantification). The patient being
      asked to differentiate the characteristic of different
      textures
    - Graphesthesia (recognition).

Two-point discrimination   A specialist tool provided with the
Rivermead Assessment of Somatosensory Performance (Fig. 23.5)
provides a standardized tool for testing, however if this is unavail-
able, two paper clips can be used.

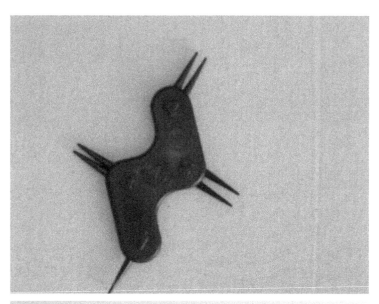

Figure 23.5 Tool for testing two-point discrimination (RASP).

1. The therapist should hold the tool against the patient's skin with constant gentle pressure over the palmar surface of the hand and fingers.
2. Randomly apply one point or two points of the tool (5 mm, 4 mm, 3 mm apart), starting with the greater distance first. The normal range for two-point discrimination on the finger pads is 2–4 mm and for the palm 8–15 mm.
3. The patient is asked to report whether they feel either one point or two points.
4. Record the distances at which the patient is able to discriminate two points. This is easily documented on a diagram of the hand.

Graphesthesia

1. The therapist uses a blunt object to draw a number or letter onto the patient's palm.
2. The patient is asked to identify the number/letter.

TACTILE – DEEP TOUCH/PRESSURE

The therapist should follow the assessment procedure as for light touch but should use the blunt end of a neurotip as the instrument for producing the stimulus of pressure (Fig. 23.6) or a

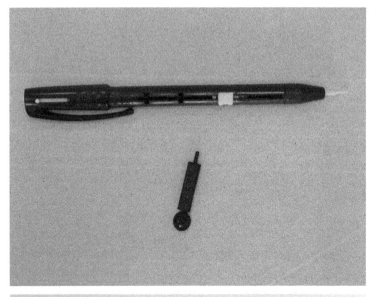

Figure 23.6 Tools for testing pressure (pressure pen and neurotip).

pressure pen, which gives a better standardization of application (Fig. 23.6). As the Pacinian corpuscles are rapid adapting receptors the neurotip should be placed on and off rather than be applied continuously.

Touch pressure threshold
Using the pressure pen, various standardized levels of pressure can be evaluated so assessing the ability of quantification.

 Caution
Healthy and Safety (Infection control) – Cotton wool balls and neurotips should be discarded after use with one patient.

PAIN (PIN PRICK)
The therapist should follow the assessment procedure as for light touch but should use the sharp end of a neurotip as the instrument for producing the stimulus of pain (Fig. 23.7). Note: Be very careful not to pierce the skin! Using the tip at a 45° angle is advised.

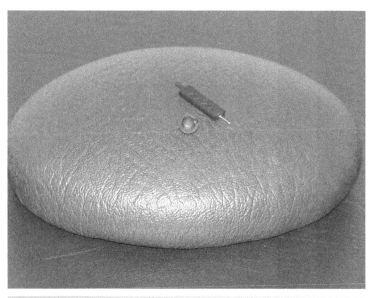
Figure 23.7 Tool for testing pain sensation (pin prick).

Sharp and blunt

This technique assesses the ability of quantification related to different characteristics of pain and is carried out using the sharp and blunt end of a neurotip (Figs 23.6, 23.7).

1. The therapist randomly applies the sharp or blunt stimulus to the test area to avoid using a pattern that may be predictable.
2. The patient is asked to report if the stimulus is 'sharp or blunt'
3. In theory, this tests the ability to differentiate fast and slow pain (quantification).

TEMPERATURE (HEAT AND NON-NOXIOUS COLD)

The therapist should follow the assessment procedure as for light touch but should use thermo controlled test tubes, one cold (6–10°C) and one hot (44–48°C) as the instruments for producing the stimulus of heat and non-noxious cold (Fig. 23.8). This procedure should test for temperature awareness of both heat and cold separately and also the ability to discriminate between the two (is this hot or cold?).

PROPRIOCEPTION

There are a few methods by which proprioception can be assessed. As traditionally these techniques are carried out with the patients

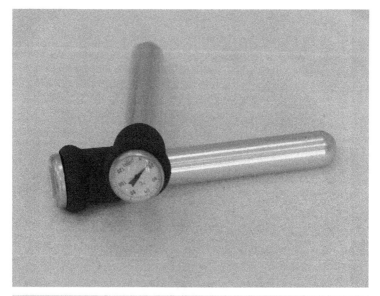

Figure 23.8 Tool for testing temperature.

eyes closed, excluding our sense of vision, a more accurate description of what is being assessed would be joint position sense and movement sense.

Mirroring

Patient   The patient may be sitting or supine.
Therapist

1. Explain and demonstrate the procedure.
2. Ask the patient to close their eyes.
3. The therapist places *and holds* one limb into a set position (Fig. 23.9).
4. The patient is requested to copy the position with the opposite limb and the therapist makes a judgement on the accuracy of the response (Fig. 23.9).
5. An inaccurate response may indicate a deficit of joint position sense.

Clinical hints and tips

For patients with a primarily unilateral dysfunction such as CVA, the therapist should place the affected limb into the position to be copied. This allows the patient an attempt to copy using the unaffected limb, which has no motor dysfunction.

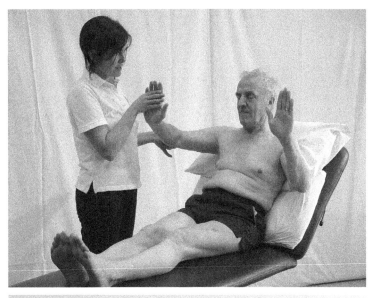

Figure 23.9 Testing for proprioception (mirroring).

However, there are several shortcomings with this method:

- It requires a certain level of motor ability in the limb being moved by the patient, therefore motor ability is being assessed simultaneously.
- In the case of conditions which present with bilateral dysfunction, such as multiple sclerosis, the test may be inaccurate and invalid as accurate assessment is not possible.
- It simultaneously assesses multiple joints.
- It allows for the assessment of position sense but not movement sense.

Specific joint position sense and movement sense testing

Patient   Supine will make assessment of both upper limbs and lower limbs more convenient.

Therapist

1. Explain and demonstrate the procedure to the patient.
2. Establishing a communication system in layman's terms is vital to the success of this method. For example, if the positions to be assessed are elbow flexion and extension, the terms used by the patient could be 'bent' (for flexion) and 'straight' (for extension). This should be clarified and agreed to prior to testing each joint.
3. Ask the patient to close their eyes.
4. The therapist places the joint being assessed in the extreme of *one position* (e.g. full elbow flexion) and holds it still (Fig. 23.10).

Clinical hints and tips

Hand hold – Whenever possible, the therapist should attempt to (a) position the patient so that the movement being assessed is gravity eliminated and (b) use a hand grip at the sides of the joint (Fig. 23.9). This will minimize the cues given to the patient through handling, making the findings more accurate.

---

5. The patient is asked to indicate the joint position (e.g. if the elbow is bent or straight).
6. This procedure should be repeated for both extremes of the same movement (e.g. full elbow flexion and extension).
7. If a deficit is suspected, additional detailed information may be gathered to assist in analysis of the problem:
   - Gross position sense. The therapist makes large changes in the position. The patient being asked is the elbow 'more bent' or 'more straight'?

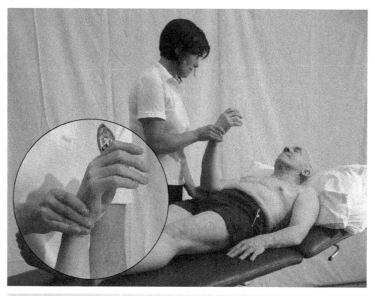

Figure 23.10 Testing for proprioception (individual joints).

- Fine position sense. The therapist makes small changes in the position and asks the patient is the elbow 'more bent' or 'more straight'?
8. Movement sense. The therapist should move the body segment and simultaneously ask the patient is the elbow 'bending' or 'straightening'? This should also be tested using large and small ranges of movement.

 Clinical hints and tips
The therapist should always assess both position and movement sense as they are derived from different sensory receptors.

9. The procedure should then be repeated for all joints and at least one direction of movement at each joint.

Stereognosis

1. The therapist places a familiar object in the patient's hand allowing manipulation of the object.
2. The patient is requested to identify the object with eyes closed.

RECORDING

A body chart provides a clear and time efficient way of representing most of the sensory findings:

- Light touch/pressure
- Pain/temperature
- Proprioception.

It is usual to record only the existing deficits, which are marked on the corresponding position of the body chart. A key indicating the symbols used to identify different modalities is advisable. Awareness, discrimination and quantification can be added as appropriate, as long as the chart remains legible. See the body chart for pain (S3.29) as an example.

Recognition by graphesthesia and stereognosis can be recorded as intact, impaired or absent. Of course a text description of the above is also perfectly acceptable.

Example

Sensory testing Light touch/pressure and temperature/pain are fully intact.

Gross positional and movement sense (proprioception) is intact throughout, however fine positional sense is reduced in left hand and two-point discrimination is increased to 8–10 mm on the left finger pads. Stereognosis is poor with left hand.

ANALYSIS

Sensory deficits may have wide ranging implications for the neurologically impaired patient from potential soft tissue damage because of lack of awareness, poor balance and falls and reduced fine finger function. Therefore, it is important for the therapist to understand the specific sensory deficit of the patient and the implications it may be having for movement and function. There is also some evidence to support the success of sensory retraining following CVA (Schabrun and Hillier 2009) and therefore accuracy in assessment is paramount.

From the above example, reduced finger joint position sense and two-point discrimination of the left hand may result in reduced fine finger function and grip. This will have greater implications if the patient is left handed. The poor stereognosis may be a reflection of the former, rather than a sensory integration problem but this would have to be explored further.

 OUTCOME MEASURES

RESEARCH

- KinCom (IsoKinetic International, Harrison, TN) can be used to quantify proprioception.
- American Spinal Injury Association score (ASIA). ASIA produces a score based on a coding system (0 = absent; 1 = abnormal; 2 = normal) (Bromley 2006). This system is widely used in spinal cord injuries where the dermatome distribution is tested but has less relevance in conditions such as CVA, multiple sclerosis and Parkinson's disease, where testing in this specific distribution is not necessary.
- Rivermead Assessment of Somatosensory Performance (RASP). The RASP provides a standardized quantifiable assessment of somatosensory impairments. A score is calculated for specified regions of the body and it has been validated for the CVA population (Winward et al. 2002). Precise instructions are included with the tool.

CLINICAL

- The Nottingham Sensory Assessment
- Rivermead Assessment of Somatosensory Performance
- ASIA score.

REFERENCES AND FURTHER READING

Blennerhassett JM, Matyas TA, Carey LM: Impaired discrimination of surface friction contributes to pinch grip deficit after stroke, *Neurorehabilitation and Neural Repair* 213:263–272, 2007.

Bromley I: *Tetraplegia and paraplegia: a guide for physiotherapists*, ed 6, Edinburgh, 2006, Churchill Livingstone.

Busse M, Tyson SF: How many body locations need to be tested when assessing sensation after stroke? An investigation of redundancy in the Rivermead Assessment of Somatosensory Performance, *Clinical Rehabilitation* 231: 91–95, 2009.

Campbell M: *Rehabilitation for traumatic brain injury: physical therapy practice in context*, Edinburgh, 2000, Churchill Livingstone.

Cassiopeia F, Okun MS: Origins of the sensory examination in neurology, *Seminars in Neurology* 22:399–408, 2002.

Collins DF, Refshauge KM, Todd G, et al: Cutaneous receptors contribute to kinesthesia at the index finger elbow and knee, *Journal of Neurophysiology* 94: 1699–1706, 2005.

Fang Y, Chen X, Li H, et al: A study on additional early physiotherapy after stroke and factors affecting functional recovery, *Clinical Rehabilitation* 176:608–617, 2003.

Fess EE: Assessment of the upper extremity: instrumentation criteria, *Occupational Therapy Practice* 1:1–11, 1990.

Forsaa EB, Larsen JP, Wentzel-Larsen T, et al: Predictors and course of health related quality of life in Parkinson's disease, *Movement Disorders* 23:1420–1427, 2008.

Juri C, Rodriguez-Oroz M, Obeso JA: The pathophysiological basis of sensory disturbances in Parkinson's disease, *Journal of Neurologic Science* 289:60–65, 2009.

Kandel ER, Schwartz JH, Jessell TM: *Principles of neural science*, ed 4, New York, 2000, McGraw-Hill.

Proske U, Gandevia SC: The kinesthetic senses, *Journal of Physiology* 587:4139–4146, 2009.

Rahman S, Griffin HJ, Quinn NP: Quality of life in Parkinson's disease: the relative importance of the symptoms, *Movement Disorders* 23:1428–1434, 2008.

Riemann BL, Lephart SM: The sensorimotor system, part I: the physiologic basis of functional joint stability, *Journal of Athletic Training* 37:71–79, 2002a.

Riemann BL, Lephart SM: The sensorimotor system, part II: the role of proprioception in motor control and functional joint stability, *Journal of Athletic Training* 37:80–84, 2002b.

Schabrun SM, Hillier S: Evidence for the retraining of sensation after stroke: a systematic review, *Clinical Rehabilitation* 231:27–39, 2009.

Smith JL, Crawford M, Proske U, et al: Signals of motor command bias joint position sense in the presence of feedback from proprioceptors, *Journal of Applied Physiology* 106:950–958, 2009.

Sturnieks DL, Wright JR, Fitzpatrick RC: Detection of simultaneous movement at two human arm joints, *Journal of Physiology* 585:833–842, 2007.

Tyson SF, Hanley M, Chillala J, et al: Sensory loss in hospital-admitted people with stroke: characteristics associated factors and relationship with function, *Neurorehabilitation and Neural Repair* 222:166–172, 2008.

Widerstrom-Noga EG, Duncan R, Felipe-Cuervo E, et al: Assessment of the impact of pain and impairments associated with spinal cord injuries, *Archives of Physical Medicine and Rehabilitation* 83:395–404, 2002.

Winward CE, Halligan PW, Wade DT: The Rivermead Assessment of Somatosensory Performance RASP: standardization and reliability data, *Clinical Rehabilitation* 16:523–533, 2002.

Zia S, Cody F, O'Boyle D: Joint position sense is impaired in Parkinson's disease, *Annals of Neurology* 47:218–228, 2000.

Dermatomes

WHAT IS A DERMATOME?

A dermatome is defined as the area of skin supplied by one spinal nerve root level. There are 31 pairs of spinal nerves leaving the spinal cord (S2.13) and each one supplies a different area of skin. Therefore the skin supplied by all the individual spinal nerve roots ultimately produces a dermatome map that represents the entire body (Fig. 24.1).

Caution

Dermatome maps vary widely between individuals and the boundaries of each dermatome may also overlap within one person.

WHY DO I NEED TO ASSESS DERMATOMES?

Assessing a dermatome gives information related to nerve integrity, in other words whether the nerve pathway from the skin to the spinal cord is intact. Knowledge of the cutaneous supply of both the spinal nerve root (dermatome) and the peripheral nerve allows the therapist to differentiate between lesions of each (Petty 2006). For example, a sensory loss of the area over the deltoid

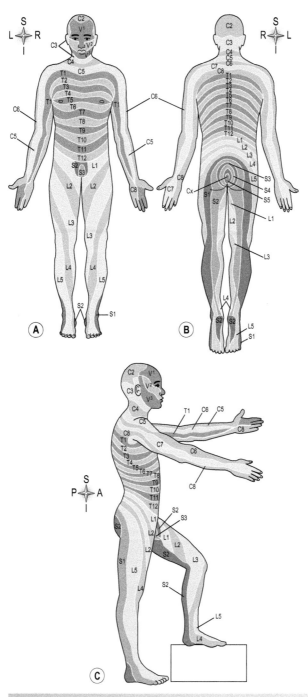

Figure 24.1 (A–C) Dermatome map.

muscle at the shoulder is identified as dermatome C_5. The same area of skin is also part of the sensory distribution of the radial nerve (posterior cutaneous nerve of the arm $C_{5/6/7/8}$ T_1). It is therefore likely, but not certain that the lesion is at the level of the spinal nerve root because a lesion of the peripheral nerve is likely to be more extensive. Accurate diagnosis is only possible with knowledge of anatomy and accurate assessment.

Caution

A sensory loss related to a single dermatome may be indicative of a lesion at the spinal nerve root **but** must be confirmed by a similar finding for that particular root level for myotomes (S3.31) and reflexes (S3.22).

In terms of neurologically impaired patients, the clinical presentation of any sensory loss *only* requires assessment using a dermatome distribution when there is involvement of either the spinal cord specifically or the peripheral nervous system, e.g. in spinal cord injury (SCI) and Guillain–Barré syndrome (GBS). As neither of these pathologies affects the spinal nerve root in isolation, dermatome testing is *less clinically useful as a diagnostic tool, however it is a very useful way of mapping the sensory loss.* The map produced gives the therapist a highly relevant outcome measure by which the extent and level of sensory loss can first be estimated and then re-evaluated. This is especially important in recovering conditions such as GBS and in SCI, where a rising level of sensory loss may reflect a serious deterioration of the injury.

HOW DO I ASSESS A DERMATOME?

PATIENT

To complete a dermatome assessment, the therapist needs to access the patient's skin over the trunk, upper and lower limbs, both anteriorly and posteriorly. This will require a change of position. For the patient's comfort the therapist could start the assessment in supine and move to prone.

THERAPIST

1. The therapist can test various sensations.
   - Light touch (cotton wool) (S3.23)
   - Deep touch/pressure (pressure pen) (S3.23)
   - Pain **or** temperature (neurotip at 45° or heat/non-noxious cold temperature device) (S3.23, 29).

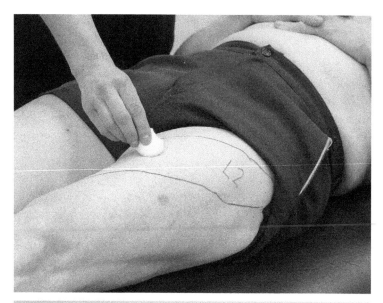

Figure 24.2 Testing a dermatome for light touch.

2. These sensations are mapped using the dermatome distribution map (Fig. 24.1). However, as each dermatome originates from a single spinal cord level the dermatomes of consecutive levels tend to overlap making the ability to differentiate between different levels close to the spine (trunk) almost impossible. Therefore the larger, more distal portion of each dermatome is used for testing during the assessment (Fig. 24.2).

3. The same procedure is used to test for all sensations with the implement for testing changing accordingly. Light touch is described as an example.

4. Explain the procedure to the patient and check their understanding upon an unaffected area of skin.

5. Ask them to close their eyes.

6. Identify a dermatome to test (without telling the patient) and use the cotton wool to dab the centre of that dermatome (Fig. 24.2).

Clinical hints and tips

Dermatomes overlap, therefore your assessment will be more accurate if you (a) dab one spot rather than dragging across the skin and (b) dab the centre of the dermatome being tested.

7. Compare the same dermatome on the left and right side of the body.
8. Repeat the procedure using a different dermatome.
9. Randomize the applications to avoid the patient being able to predict a pattern of testing. The therapist then maps out any area of altered or diminished sensation.

   Are they able to feel anything? No, anaesthesia (loss of sensation) could indicate a complete lesion of the spinal root pathway.

   What do they feel? Any tingling or burning sensations? Paraesthesia or abnormal sensation indicates abnormal transmission along the nerve pathway (S3.23). This could occur as a result of any condition which affects the transmission of action potentials along the neuron. For example, nerve compression, inflammation, infection, virus, reduced circulation or demyelination. Tactile hyperaesthesia or excessive sensation could be a result of peripheral sensitization (S3.29).

   Is any sensory loss confined to the dermatome? Yes would implicate a single nerve root. However, if the loss is wider, more than one nerve root could be involved or the lesion may not be specific to the nerve root itself.

   Does it feel the same both sides? No. Assuming a unilateral pathology the unaffected side can be used as a normative baseline to assess any abnormalities. In conditions where bilateral lesions are suspected this is not valid and the therapist should compare to an expected norm.

RECORDING

Record any loss of sensation or abnormal sensation for each dermatome. Traditionally, the findings are recorded on a body chart with shaded areas used to represent areas of skin with abnormal sensation. Different sensations will require different shading design and hence a key to ensure the findings are clear to another clinician. This mapping should be completed accurately so that any increase in the area (condition worsening) or decrease in the area (condition improving) can be identified.

ANALYSIS

If the tests indicate a specific area of loss, a spinal nerve root deficit may be suspected and may be confirmed by comparing any abnormal findings for the same root level for myotome testing and reflexes. If the loss is widespread the lesion is likely to be more generalized to the peripheral nervous system and can be used to identify the extent and level of a lesion.

OUTCOME MEASURE

RESEARCH AND CLINICAL
- ASIA score (S3.23)
- Dermatome testing is viewed as an outcome measure to be used as an ongoing tool for evaluation.

REFERENCE
Petty NJ: *Neuromusculoskeletal examination and assessment: a handbook for therapists*, ed 3, Edinburgh, 2006, Churchill Livingstone.

Trunk stability

WHAT IS TRUNK STABILITY?

The terms trunk/central and spinal stability are synonymous and are used interchangeably in clinical practice. Core stability is the equivalent lay term. In essence, trunk stability is a reflection of an individual's postural control, the ability to orientate and stabilize the body using appropriate balance strategies and responses (Raine et al. 2009). As such, trunk stability is an essential core component of balance, the ability to maintain the centre of mass (COM) within the base of support (BOS) (S3.32) and functional activities, by which it provides proximal stability to allow for the coordinated free movement of the limbs and head (Brown 2006; Massion et al. 2004). Trunk stability is also important in controlling and supporting the spinal segments, so reducing the stresses upon soft tissue structures and helping to avoid injury and pain.

Trunk stability mainly incorporates muscle activation related to the trunk, head/neck and proximal limb girdles. However, it is also described as a muscular 'box' that is made up of the diaphragm superiorly, the pelvic floor and gluteal muscles inferiorly, the abdominals anteriorly and the back extensors posteriorly. The therapist should remain aware of the 'box' as a whole in terms of strategies they may use to facilitate treatment (through contraction of the pelvic floor) and tricks that the patient may use to achieve false stability (breath holding).

This section will focus upon the core trunk muscles which are commonly divided into two groups according to their functional anatomy (Bergmark 1989):

THE GLOBAL STABILIZERS
This group includes:

- External obliques
- Internal obliques
- Rectus abdominus
- Erector spinae.

These muscles are anatomically superficial and their action does not have an influence at a segmental level. They are composed primarily of Type IIx (fast glycolytic fibres) muscle fibres which can generate larger forces but are fast fatiguing. The function of the global stabilizers is primarily trunk movement, although they do contribute to general trunk stability.

THE LOCAL STABILIZERS
This group includes:

- Multifidus (MT)
- Transversus abdominus (TAb)
- Inferior fibres of internal oblique (IOf)

These muscles are anatomically deep and have attachments to each individual spinal vertebra. This allows them to act at a segmental level (between adjacent vertebrae) providing a strong basis for trunk stability. The local stabilizers are composed primarily of Type I (slow oxidative fibres) muscle fibres, which produce low forces but are fatigue resistant. These muscles therefore function as postural muscles. They also have smaller motor units which are easily activated due to their low neural threshold and therefore tend to be recruited first (Henneman principle) during functional activities. In theory, this means that the local stabilizers are activated prior to the surrounding global muscles which have larger motor units. This pre-setting of trunk stability is crucial in providing a stable base upon which limb movement can be based and may be part of an anticipatory response to a perceived COM displacement (MacDonald et al. 2006). The anticipatory activation will be built into a learned movement plan.

The anatomical and physiological features of the local muscle stabilizers make them perfectly adapted to perform their specific trunk stability function, however the nervous system also influences the fine control of these muscles. The force of contraction required to provide segmental stability is estimated to be 3% of maximum contraction (Cholewicki and McGill 1996). As anti-gravity postural muscles, this background level of activity is controlled by the vestibular and reticular systems (S2.10).

The balance of activity between the abdominal (TAb/IOf) and back extensor (MT) pair is vital in terms of the level and timing of activation. A neutral position of the pelvis and lumbar spine is considered to be highly correlated with the co-contraction of this muscle pair (O'Sullivan 2006). In postures of either anterior pelvic tilt with lumbar spine hyperextension or posterior tilt with lumbar spine flexion the local muscles are switched off and over time become deconditioned (O'Sullivan 2006). This is highly relevant in a population of neurologically impaired patients who often spend many hours sitting in poor postures in inadequate seating.

WHY DO I NEED TO ASSESS TRUNK STABILITY?

Trunk instability results in less efficient movement, a limited ability to explore the environment (Cristea et al. 2003) and demands compensatory muscle activity to maintain an upright position. The latter may present as abnormal fixation of the trunk or, in extreme cases, excessive use of the upper limbs, and leads to effortful movement for the individual. Poor trunk stability resulting in deviations in posture may also cause abnormal stresses and potential damage to soft tissue structures leading to pain and further functional loss. Often rehabilitation focuses on improving general trunk stability without specific attention to the interaction between the local and global stabilizers. More focus on segmental stability initially may have the potential to improve the movement sequences and the functional outcome for the individual.

In a neurologically impaired patient, poor trunk stability has been linked with a poor functional outcome in multiple sclerosis

(Lanzetta et al. 2004), cerebrovascular accident (CVA) (Hsieh et al. 2002) and Parkinson's disease (PD) (Dibble and Lange 2006; Nardone and Schieppati 2006).

In CVA, trunk instability has also been linked with poor postural control in standing (Palmer et al. 1996; Slijper et al. 2002) and in sitting (Dickstein et al. 2004) and is viewed as a negative prognostic indicator for recovery. Proprioception (position sense) (Mergner et al. 2003; Peterka 2002) and reduced strength (Karatas et al. 2004) in the trunk have been found to be causal in CVA (Ryerson et al. 2008) and in PD (Vaugoyeau et al. 2007).

HOW DO I ASSESS TRUNK STABILITY?

OBSERVATION DURING FUNCTIONAL ACTIVITIES

Patient

Any trunk instability may have already been noted during the second section of the objective assessment (S3.18). However, as the demands on trunk stability appear to be task specific the therapist should ensure they have investigated a range of functional activities.

Therapist

The therapist observes the patient during a functional activity.

How much postural sway is observed in a static position? The normal excursion of postural sway should be very small, occurring in response to the action of gravity and breathing perturbations. If the movements are large, this could indicate trunk instability.

Does this postural sway deteriorate with eyes closed? This could indicate insufficient sensory feedback as a cause of instability.

Do they have difficulty achieving tasks using their upper limbs? They may be using their arms to fix and therefore will be reluctant to use them during functional activities.

Do they lose balance during tasks? Yes, this may indicate trunk instability.

Is there excessive trunk movement when:
  Both upper limbs are raised?
  Performing any functional activity? Yes, these may indicate trunk instability.
    Do they have difficulty with lower limb placement during swing phase? Scissoring may reflect the inability to place the foot

accurately because of an unstable trunk in contralateral stance.

Do they use any compensatory fixation? This may involve limbs or fixation/excessive stiffness through the trunk and may indicate trunk instability or a lack confidence to move.

ASSESSMENT OF THE LOCAL MUSCLE STABILIZERS

Patient

Initially in terms of patient safety, it is wise to begin assessing the patient in a sitting position. However, for higher level patients, a further assessment when standing may also be pertinent.

Therapist: observe and palpate

1. Initially the patient's position should reflect their posture of choice, in order for the therapist to assess the trunk stabilizers under normal circumstances.
2. Ask the patient to perform a limb movement in order to challenge the trunk stabilizers. This could include one arm being lifted (shoulder flexion or abduction), two arms being raised or one leg being lifted (hip flexion or abduction). The amount the limb is moved will depend on the ability of the individual. In some cases the ability to raise a hand 2 inches may be very challenging.
3. Observe and then palpate the local stabilizers to evaluate the state of contraction.
   a. Multifidus (MT): Palpate for MT just medial to the posterior superior iliac spine (PSIS) (Fig. 25.1).
   b. Transversus abdominus (TAb): Palpate 1 inch medially and 1 inch inferiorly from the anterior superior iliac spine (ASIS) (Fig. 25.2).

Clinical hints and tips

Although MT is found at all levels of the vertebral column it is at its thickest in the cervical and lumbar areas and it is superficial from level L_3 down.

Anatomically, in cadavers, the TAb and IOf muscles have been found to be fused at this palpation point (Marshall and Murphy 2003). The therapist should be aware they are palpating both muscles, however this is deemed clinically acceptable when considering that they are also functionally compatible.

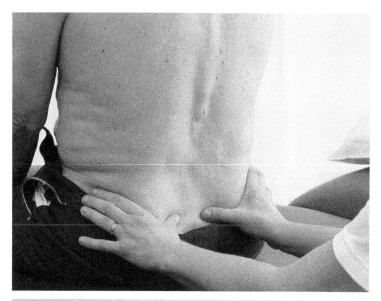

Figure 25.1 Palpation for multifidus.

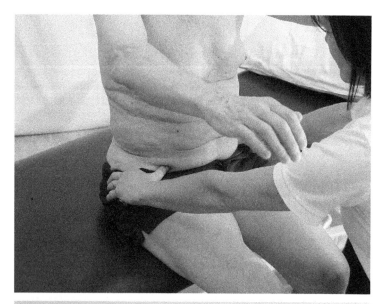

Figure 25.2 Palpation for transversus abdominus.

Can they activate the local muscle stabilizers during the task?
Or do they primarily use a global muscle contraction to gain
stability.

Can they maintain the contraction? If they can recruit the local
stabilizers, do they have good muscle endurance? If not, this
may lead to trunk instability linked to muscle weakness or
fatigue.

Is there appropriate co-contraction of the local stabilizers? There
should be simultaneous contraction of MT and TAb but the
degree of contraction of each will be dictated by the task
requirements. During a unilateral limb movement the contralateral pair of stabilizers (MT and TAb) should contract more
strongly and in a bilateral task there should be symmetry of
contraction.

Clinical hints and tips

During a simple bilateral arm raise through shoulder flexion the
COM is displaced forward and therefore stabilizer activity is
greatest in the back extensors. During a unilateral leg lift
through hip flexion, the COM is initially displaced backwards
and therefore the greatest stabilizer activity is recorded in the
abdominals to maintain the alignment of the pelvis.

Do they activate the local stabilizers prior to limb movement? This
is evidence of an anticipatory contraction. Poor sequencing
of muscle recruitment may result in trunk instability and the
need for compensatory strategies. However, in electromyo-
graphical (EMG) studies the anticipatory response is a fraction
of a second and is unlikely to be identifiable in practice.
Appreciation of a simultaneous activation is more realistic.

Do they use compensatory strategies? Common examples include
breath holding, over use of the global stabilizers, excessive use
of the shoulder elevators or hip adductors/flexors. These are
strategies used to provide false stability.

Therapist: realign pelvis/lumbar spine

1. If no muscle contraction can be palpated with the patient in
their posture of choice (Fig. 25.3) then the therapist should
try altering the alignment of the patient's pelvis/lumbar spine.
A neutral alignment of the pelvis and lumbar spine is correlated
with the preferential recruitment of the local stabilizer muscles
(O'Sullivan et al. 2006).

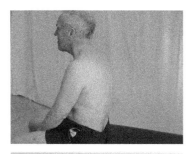

Figure 25.3 Posture of choice (sitting).

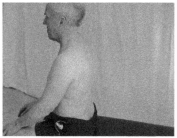

Figure 25.4 Neutral pelvis and lumbar spine (sitting).

2. The therapist should instruct or facilitate the patient towards a more neutral alignment (Fig. 25.4).
3. Reassess as for observation and palpation.

 Clinical hints and tips
Any soft tissue shortening or pain in the region of the pelvis and lumbar spine will limit the individual's ability to attain a neutral alignment. Perfect is rarely possible but a movement towards neutral may still be beneficial.

Therapist: assessment of individual muscle components
   If the patient is still unable to recruit the appropriate muscles with the pelvis/lumbar spine in a neutral alignment then the therapist should evaluate the patient's ability to activate the local muscle components individually.
Transversus abdominus (TAb)
   a. To evaluate TAb, use crook lying (i.e. supine with knees bent up to 90°) (Fig. 25.5). The aim is to encourage an isolated contraction of TAb through the alignment of a neutral pelvis and lumbar spine.
   b. The instruction to the patient will be dependent on the initial position adopted by the individual. A patient who adopts crook lying with an anteriorly tilted pelvis and extended lumbar spine needs an instruction such as 'flatten your back' or 'push your back down onto the bed' or 'pull your belly button in'. Whereas a patient who initially presents in posterior pelvic tilt and lumbar spine flexion will need to raise their back towards neutral.

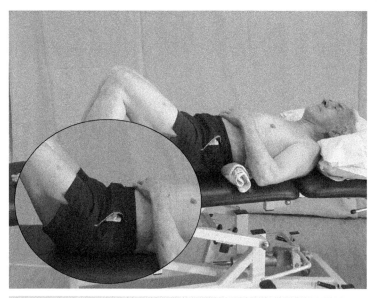

Figure 25.5 Modified crook lying.

    c. A rolled towel (2 inches thick) placed under the patient's back, at waist level (Fig. 25.5), allows for a larger movement by which to achieve neutral making the task easier for the patient to comprehend and feel.

    d. Initially the therapist may ask the patient just to tighten these muscles (an isometric contraction).

    e. If an isometric contraction can be initiated limb movements may be added in the same position to assess whether the contraction can be maintained during a challenge.

    f. The therapist should then return to the observation and palpation assessment protocol and re-test.

Multifidus (MT)

    a. To evaluate MT, use sitting. The aim is to focus on a contraction of MT through a neutral alignment of pelvis and lumbar spine.

    b. From upright sitting the therapist instructs and/or facilitates a release of the lumbar spine into flexion. This allows for a larger movement to achieve neutral and is therefore easier for the patient to comprehend and feel (Fig. 25.6).

    c. The patient is then guided towards a neutral sitting posture using facilitation. Simultaneously, the patient should attempt

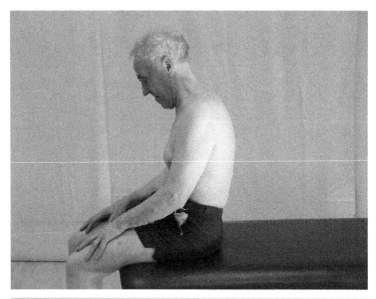

Figure 25.6 Preparation: Release of lumbar spine.

to activate the appropriate muscle while being given immediate accurate verbal feedback on the accuracy of recruitment from the therapist.
d. If an isolated contraction of MT is achieved, limb movements may be added in the same position to assess whether the contraction can be challenged.
e. The therapist should then return to the observation and palpation assessment protocol and re-test.

Caution
Remember that the local stabilizers need only work with low force to achieve segmental stability, therefore be careful not to over motivate the patient.

RECORDING

A simple heading and text description of all the therapist's findings is acceptable, or notation with a key on a body chart.

Example Trunk stability: patient presents with exaggerated postural sway during all upper limb activities. Postural sway increases with eyes closed. Patient is able to isolate both local stabilizers appropriately in sitting with effort and focused attention. Muscle tone in the trunk appears normal however proprioception is reduced.

ANALYSIS

The findings from an assessment of trunk stability should be considered in relation to other assessment tools (S3.19–34) and especially postural control/balance as the two are highly integrated. Analysis and synthesis of all this information may allow the therapist to predict a possible cause of the trunk instability.

In terms of the above example, the cause of the increased postural sway is likely to be altered sensory feedback (proprioception). This is reinforced when vision is withdrawn and the patient presents with an increase in sway.

OUTCOME MEASURE

RESEARCH
- EMG

CLINICAL
- Trunk control test
- Trunk Impairment Scale.

REFERENCES AND FURTHER READING
Bergmark A: Stability of the lumbar spine: a study in mechanical engineering, *Acta Orthopaedica Scandinavica* 230(Suppl):20–24, 1989.

Brown TD: Getting to the core of the matter, *Strengthening and Conditioning Journal* 282:1524–1604, 2006.

Cholewicki J, McGill S: Mechanical stability of the in vivo lumbar spine: implications for injury and chronic low back pain, *Clinical Biomechanics* 11:1–15, 1996.

Cristea MC, Mitnitski AB, Feldman AG, et al: Interjoint coordination dynamics during reaching in stroke, *Experimental Brain Research* 1513:289–300, 2003.

Dibble LE, Lange M: Predicting falls in individuals with Parkinson disease: a reconsideration of clinical balance measures, *Journal of Neurologic Physical Therapy* 30:60–67, 2006.

Dickstein R, Sheffi S, Markovici E: Anticipatory postural adjustment in selected trunk muscles in post stroke hemiparetic patients, *Archives of Physical Medicine and Rehabilitation* 85:228–234, 2004.

Hsieh CL, Sheu CF, Hsueh IP, et al: Trunk control as an early predictor of comprehensive activities of daily living function in stroke patients, *Stroke* 33:2626–2630, 2002.

Karatas M, Cetin N, Bayramoglu M, et al: Trunk muscle strength in relation to balance and functional disability in unihemispheric stroke patients, *American Journal of Physical Medicine and Rehabilitation* 83:81–87, 2004.

Lanzetta D, Cattaneo D, Pellegatta D, et al: Trunk control in unstable sitting posture during functional activities in healthy subjects and patients with multiple sclerosis, *Archives of Physical Medicine and Rehabilitation* 85:279–283, 2004.

MacDonald DA, Moseley GL, Hodges PW: The lumbar multifidus: does the evidence support clinical belief? *Manual Therapy* 11:254–263, 2006.

Marshall P, Murphy B: The validity and reliability of surface EMG to assess the neuromuscular response of the abdominal muscles to rapid limb movement, *Journal of Electromyography and Kinesiology* 13:477–489, 2003.

Massion J, Alexandrov A, Frolov A: Why and how are posture and movement coordinated? *Progress in Brain Research* 1432:13–27, 2004.

Mergner T, Mauer C, Peterka RA: Multisensory posture control model of human upright stance, *Progress in Brain Research* 142:189–201, 2003.

Nardone A, Schieppati M: Balance in Parkinson's disease under static and dynamic conditions, *Movement Disorders* 21:1515–1520, 2006.

O'Sullivan PB, Dankearts W, Burnett AF, et al: Effect of different upright sitting postures on spinal-pelvic curvature and trunk muscle activation in a pain free population, *Spine* 3119: E707–E712, 2006.

Palmer E, Downes L, Ashby P: Associated postural adjustments are impaired by a lesion of the cortex, *Neurology* 46:471–475, 1996.

Peterka JR: Sensorimotor integration in human postural control, *Journal of Neurophysiology* 883:1097–1118, 2002.

Raine S, Meadows L, Lynch-Ellerington M: *Bobath concept theory and clinical practice in neurological rehabilitation*, Oxford, 2009, Wiley Blackwell.

Ryerson S, Byl NN, Brown DA, et al: Altered trunk position sense and its relation to balance functions in people post-stroke, *Journal of Neurologic Physical Therapy* 321:14–20, 2008.

Slijper H, Latash M, Rao N, et al: Task specific modulation of anticipatory postural adjustments in individuals with hemiparesis, *Clinical Neurophysiology* 113:642–655, 2002.

Vaugoyeau M, Viel S, Assaiante C, et al: Impaired vertical postural control and proprioceptive integration deficits in Parkinson's disease, *Neuroscience* 146:852–863, 2007.

Coordination

 WHAT IS COORDINATION?

Successful movement involves the complex coordination of multiple joints and muscles which is achieved via the appropriate sequencing, timing and grading of muscle recruitment (Shumway-Cook and Woollacott 2007; Berthier et al. 2005). Even a simple reaching task involves all levels of the central and peripheral nervous system with the integration of these sensorimotor systems occurring primarily in the cerebellum (S2.12) (Fuller 2004). Smooth accurate movement involves the interaction of hand–eye coordination, inter-limb and trunk coordination.

INCOORDINATED MOVEMENT

Incoordination presents as a lack of smooth sequenced movement which is often awkward and uneven and may involve both limb and trunk muscles. The incoordination is attributed to a loss of synergistic interplay between muscles as a result of disruption in muscle:

- Activation
- Sequencing
- Timing
- Grading.

As the control facilitating coordinated movement is highly complex and involves many nervous system structures it follows that incoordination can be a consequence of damage to any one of them. This includes:

- Cerebellum (S2.12)
- Motor cortex (S2.7)
- Basal ganglia (S2.11)
- Sensory feedback: Proprioception (S2.23) or vision (S2.10 and S3.27)
- Motor output: Altered muscle tone (S3.21) or muscle weakness (S3.30).

Ataxia

Ataxia is a term used to describe the motor incoordination presented by patients with a deficit affecting the cerebellum (S2.12) during voluntary movement. It includes symptoms such as nystagmus, reduced manual dexterity, poor balance and altered gait (Bakker et al. 2006; Ilg et al. 2008), dysarthria and dysmetria (Thoma et al. 2008). Dysmetria, is a problem with judging the distance of movement and is often referred to as intention tremor. The outcome is inaccurate movement with overshooting (hypermetria) and undershooting (hypometria) during the task. Ataxia can affect the trunk (trunk ataxia) or limbs (limb ataxia) or both, depending on whether the lesion is in midline or the cerebellar hemispheres, respectively. The incoordinated movement that is produced affects mobility, when the patient presents with a drunken swaggering gait and all other functional activities. Ataxic movement is thought to occur due to impairment in the timing and duration of muscle activation, or the magnitude and grading of force production (Ausim 2007).

 Caution

Incoordinated movement which mimics cerebellar ataxia can occur as a result of sensory loss (sensory ataxia). The causes are very different.

WHY DO I NEED TO ASSESS COORDINATION?

Incoordinated movement is often inaccurate, effortful and ultimately leads to a reduced functional outcome. This presentation is observed in many neurologically impaired patients whether the pathology affects the central or peripheral nervous system.

HOW DO I ASSESS COORDINATION?

OBSERVATION OF FUNCTIONAL TASKS

Assessment of coordination usually begins by observing the patient's ability to perform simple functional tasks (S3.18) taking note of the accuracy, speed and trajectory of movement.

The activities observed should challenge both the limbs and trunk. To identify a trunk deficit in isolation, the patient could be requested to sit unsupported with upper limbs held in a static position away from the body. Excessive movement of the trunk could indicate incoordination. However, the therapist should be mindful that there is a great deal of overlap between the concepts of trunk coordination, trunk stability (S3.25) and balance (S3.32). The therapist should also be aware that any problems with trunk coordination will also affect the accuracy of limb movements.

SIMPLE TESTS OF LIMB COORDINATION

A comparison of right and left should be made, allowing for handedness during the performance. If there is an unaffected side this should be tested first to ensure understanding of the procedure.

The patient is scored as:

5 – Normal
4 – Minimal impairment
3 – Moderate impairment
2 – Severe impairment
1 – Unable to perform (Schmitz 2001).

Finger-to-nose test

Patient   The patient is sitting.
Therapist
1. The therapist sits in front of the patient, facing them.
2. The therapist holds their finger in front of the patient at eye level (approx. arms length from the patient).

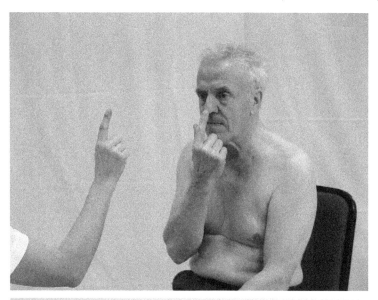

Figure 26.1 Finger–nose test.

3. With eyes *open* the patient is asked to touch their own nose with their index finger and then touch the therapist's finger (Fig. 26.1).
4. This is repeated several times and should be accomplished smoothly and easily.
5. If the performance is accurate, ask the patient to repeat the movement faster.
6. Modify the position of the therapist's finger and repeat the test, to test different planes of movement.
7. This test can be repeated with eyes closed with the patient *only touching their own nose.*

Heel–shin test

Patient Patient should be in supine on a plinth or sitting on a chair.

Therapist

1. The patient is asked to place the heel of one lower limb to touch the knee of the opposite leg.
2. The patient is requested to run the heel down the shin towards the ankle joint (Fig. 26.2). This should be accomplished smoothly and easily.

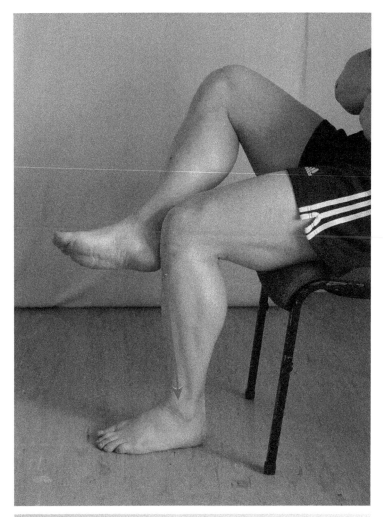

Figure 26.2 Heel–shin test.

3. If the performance is accurate this can be repeated several times with increasing speed.
4. Repeat with eyes closed.

 Caution

Patients with very poor coordination should be advised to take care during both the finger–nose and heel–shin tests to avoid any damage to eyes or the skin of the lower limb.

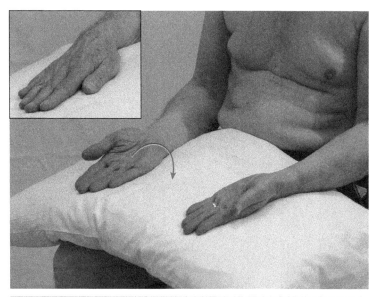

Figure 26.3 Testing for dysdiadochokinesia.

Dysdiadochokinesia

This is the inability to perform rapidly alternating movements.

Patient   Patient should be sitting.

Therapist

1. The patient should start with one hand rested on their thigh (palm down).
2. They are then asked to turn the hand over (palm up) and continue alternating between palm up and down at a reasonable speed (Fig. 26.3).
3. Repeat with the other hand.
4. This test can be modified so that the patient performs the task at 90° shoulder flexion or by alternating different opposing muscle groups around other peripheral joints (e.g. flexion and extension of the knee).

Note: Dysdiadochokinesia is commonly seen as part of ataxia (cerebellar lesion) but is also difficult to achieve for patients with hypertonia and hypotonia (S3.21).

Hand 'flip' test (inter-limb coordination)

Patient   Patient is sitting.

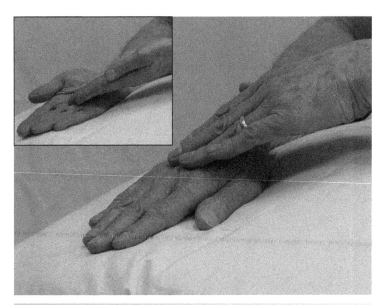

Figure 26.4 Hand 'flip' test.

Therapist

1. The patient starts with left hand palm down on their lap (the stationary hand).
2. The patient is asked to touch the back of the left hand with the anterior aspect of the fingers of the right hand (Fig. 26.4).
3. The left hand is then turned over (palm up) and the patient touches the palm with the posterior aspect of the fingers of the right hand (Fig. 26.4).
4. This is repeated several times as quickly as possible.
5. Repeat the test with the right hand stationary.
6. Repeat with eyes closed.

Other simple tests

- Drawing a circle in the air – upper or lower limb
- Hand tapping
- Foot tapping.

Is there any deviation from the expected smooth accurate movement?
Does the heel fall off the anterior part of the shin?
Is there evidence of hand slapping rather than a touch?
Does the performance deteriorate when the speed is increased?

Does the patient overshoot or undershoot the target? Yes, this is dysmetria.

Does the performance deteriorate significantly with eyes closed? If the original task was accurate this may indicate a deficit of proprioception.

Is there excessive trunk movement during the task? This could indicate trunk involvement. Sit the patient supported and re-test.

RECORDING

A simple text description of what was tested and the findings is sufficient.

Example Finger–nose test

- Left: Nothing abnormal detected (NAD)
- Right: Inaccurate and slow.

ANALYSIS

Testing coordination informs the therapist of the existence of a movement dysfunction but not about its cause. Further investigation using other objective assessment tools (S3.19–34), integrated with knowledge related to the patient's pathological condition will facilitate analysis of the causal factors.

REFERENCES AND FURTHER READING

Ausim AS: And the olive said to the cerebellum: organization and functional significance of the olivo-cerebellar system, *Neuroscientist* 13:616–626, 2007.

Bakker M, Allum JH, Visser JE, et al: Postural responses to multidirectional stance perturbations in cerebellar ataxia, *Experimental Neurology* 202:21–35, 2006.

Berthier NE, Rosenstein MT, Barto AG: Approximate optimal control as a model for motor learning, *Psychological Review* 112:329–346, 2005.

Crawford JD, Medendorp WP, Marotta JJ: Spatial transformations for eye–hand coordination, *Journal of Neurophysiology* 92110–92119, 2004.

Fuller G: *Neurological examination made easy*, ed 3, Edinburgh, 2004, Churchill Livingstone.

Ilg W, Giese MA, Gizewski ER, et al: The influence of focal cerebellar lesions on the control and adaptation of gait, *Brain* 131:2913–2927, 2008.

Johansson RS, Westling G, Bäckström A, et al: Eye–hand coordination in object manipulation, *Journal of Neuroscience* 2117:6917–6932, 2001.

Schmitz TJ: Coordination assessment. In O'Sullivan SB, Schmitz TJ, editors: *Physical rehabilitation assessment and treatment*, ed 4, Philadelphia, 2001, FA Davis.

Shumway-Cook A, Woollacott MH: *Motor control translating research into clinical practice*, ed 3, Philadelphia, 2007, Lippincott Williams and Wilkins.

Thoma P, Bellebaum C, Koch B, et al: The cerebellum is involved in reward-based reversal learning, *Cerebellum* 7:433–443, 2008.

Vision

WHAT ASPECTS OF VISION DO I NEED TO ASSESS?

Visual testing is usually completed by the medical team as part of the assessment of the cranial nerves (S2.10). Visual acuity should be assessed by an optometrist using a Snellen eye chart. However, there are aspects of vision that are simple and relevant for the therapist to assess:

VISUAL FIELDS

The input from central and peripheral visual fields (S2.10) is important in providing a complete picture of the external environment. Therefore any lesion involving the visual pathway could result in incomplete input, which may hinder functional ability. The presentation of lesions at different points along the visual pathway is shown in Table 27.1.

Clinical hints and tips
It may be useful to clarify the outcome of these lesions in conjunction with the visual pathway (see Fig. 10.1 in S2.10).

Table 27.1 Lesions of different parts of the visual pathway in terms of the visual field deficit (X indicates the area of deficit)

Lesion of the:	Left eye		Right eye		Functional outcome
	Temporal field	Nasal field	Nasal field	Temporal field	
Left optic nerve	X	X			Blind in left eye
Optic chiasma	X			X	Tunnel vision (Bitemporal hemianopia)
Left optic tract		X		X	Homonymous hemianopia
Left optic radiation		X		X	Homonymous hemianopia
Left occipital lobe		X		X	Homonymous hemianopia
Uncrossed info. from nasal fields		X	X		Binasal hemianopia

FIXING AND SCANNING

Visual acuity requires coordination between head and body movements to allow the visual stimuli to be picked up by the appropriate part of the retina. This is achieved via fixing (S2.10) and scanning (S2.10). A deficit affecting these abilities may produce poor balance and inaccurate movement during function.

WHY DO I NEED TO ASSESS THESE ASPECTS OF VISION?

Visual deficits are present in as many as 40% of patients with cerebrovascular accidents and 50% of traumatic brain injuries (Kerty 2005). Vision is important in the context of balance and movement and therefore any deficit may have a profound effect on the patient's ability to function.

HOW DO I ASSESS THESE ASPECTS OF VISION?

VISUAL FIELDS

Patient

The patient should be seated.

Therapist

1. Use a long object (such as a ruler) for testing to avoid arms being seen when reaching around in front of the patient's face.
2. The therapist should stand behind the patient. In addition it is preferable to have an assistant sitting in front of the patient to provide a visual target on which the patient can focus and from where compliance to the protocol can be evaluated.
3. Ask the patient to keep looking straight ahead at all times.
4. Ask the patient to verbalize or raise a hand when they see any change in their visual environment.
5. The therapist then starts to move the ruler from behind the patient's head in an arc towards the front of the patient's face, keeping it equidistant from the patient (Fig. 27.1).
6. If the patient acknowledges the stimuli the therapist may decide to confirm the observation by randomly keeping the ruler still and then moving it a small distance backwards and forwards. Ask the patient to report whether the ruler is still or moving.
7. Return to the start position.
8. To give a complete picture, this arc-like movement needs to be repeated for left and right sides and for upper and lower quadrants.
9. The therapist should mix up the order of testing so that the patient is unable to predict the stimuli.

Are all visual fields intact? No, there may be a deficit of the visual pathway. The normal range of the visual fields for one eye is 60° medially, 90° laterally, 50° superiorly and 70° inferiorly (Fig. 27.2). The pattern of any deficit may help diagnose the location of the lesion (Table 27.1). If this deficit is not being managed referral back to the medical team is required.

 Caution

Spatial inattention and neglect (S3.33) may present similarly and may be difficult to differentiate.

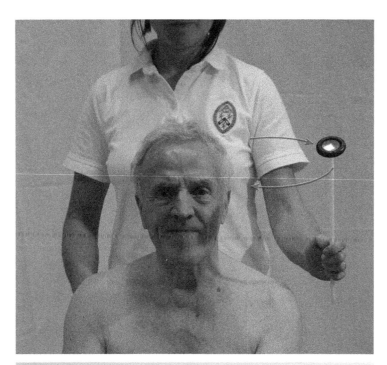

Figure 27.1 Testing visual fields.

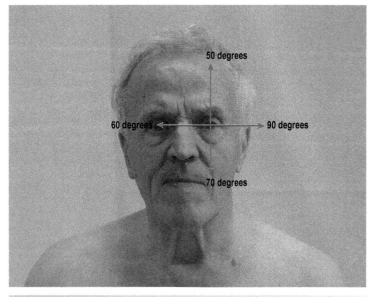

Figure 27.2 Extremes of unilateral visual field.

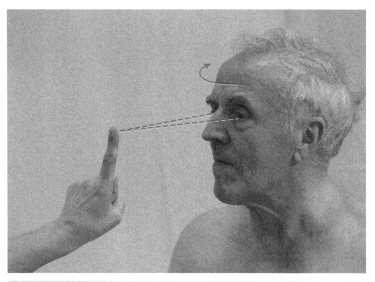

Figure 27.3 Testing visual fixing.

FIXING (FIG. 27.3)

Patient
The patient should be seated.

Therapist
1. The therapist should sit 3–6 feet in front of the patient, facing them.
2. The therapist holds their finger up in front of the patient's face, about 2 feet away from their nose.
3. Keep the finger still, the patient is requested to keep their eyes on the finger while turning their head towards the right.
4. Ask them to return to the centre and then repeat to the left.

Are they able to maintain a fixed gaze upon your finger? If not there could be a deficit of the vestibulocular reflex (VOR), implicating the vestibular system or the cranial nerve nuclei III or VI.

SCANNING (FIG. 27.4)

Patient
The patient should be seated.

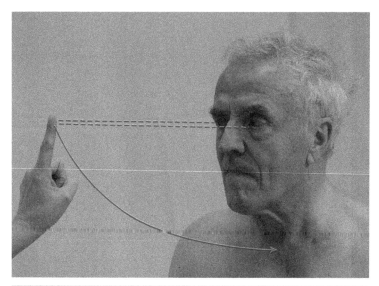

Figure 27.4 Testing visual scanning.

Therapist

1. The therapist should sit 3–6 feet in front of the patient, facing them.
2. The therapist holds their finger up in front of the patient's face.
3. The patient should keep their head facing the therapist and completely still throughout the procedure.
4. The therapist then moves their finger laterally and asks the patient to follow the course of their finger with their eyes only. Ask them to follow your finger back to the centre.
5. The therapist then needs to repeat the assessment in all six cardinal directions or in an 'H' pattern.

Are they able to scan throughout the range? If not, there may be a deficit of the cranial nerves III, IV or VI.

Is there any oscillation of the eye during the upward and lateral gaze? This could be nystagmus. This represents an incoordination of the muscles controlling the eye movements. It is often associated with ataxia (S3.26) and indicative of a cerebellum lesion.

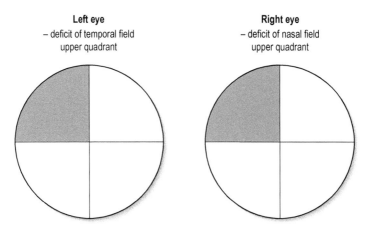

Left eye
– deficit of temporal field
upper quadrant

Right eye
– deficit of nasal field
upper quadrant

Figure 27.5 Example of recording visual fields.

RECORDING

Recording the findings for fixing and scanning could utilize a simple text description of the deficits noted. However, it may be more efficient to note any visual field deficit in a circle representing the four quadrants tested (Fig. 27.5).

Example
Visual testing:

- Fixing (VOR): Intact
- Scanning
  - To the left: Intact
  - To the right: Right eye presents with nystagmus end range of temporal field
- Visual fields (see Fig. 27.5).

REFERENCE
Kerty E: Vision rehabilitation after brain injury, *Tidsskr Nor Laegeforen* 125(2):146, 2005.

28

Range of movement

WHAT IS RANGE OF MOVEMENT (ROM)?

The function of a joint is to allow full range, friction free movement between its segments. The full range of movement (FROM) of a joint incorporates both the accessory movement (which cannot be produced in isolation by an individual) and the physiological movement.

ACTIVE PHYSIOLOGICAL MOVEMENT

The physiological movement of a joint is the active voluntary movement that a person can perform themselves. When performing an active physiological movement (AROM) there is combined involvement of the joint, muscle and motor control. Therefore these are all potential sources of dysfunction. The more common presentation is that of a reduced ROM, however instability, loss of proprioception and poor control could lead to an excessive ROM. In a neurologically impaired patient the potential causes of altered AROM include:

- Altered muscle tone (S3.21)
- Altered sensation (especially proprioception) (S3.23)
- Altered motor control (S2.7)
- Incoordination/ataxia (S3.26)
- Pain (S3.29)
- Cognitive/perceptual deficit (S3.33)
- Lack of confidence
- Soft tissue contracture
- Weakness (S3.30).

 Clinical hints and tips
Remember that AROM may also be influenced by factors such as age, gender, occupation, handedness, time of day, temperature, emotional status and other pathology.

PASSIVE PHYSIOLOGICAL MOVEMENT

A passive physiological movement (PROM) is defined as a movement within the unrestricted ROM for a segment, which is produced entirely by an external force. In the spinal joints this is referred to as a 'passive physiological intervertebral movement' (PPIVM). Although not actively involved in producing the movement, muscles and other soft tissue around the joint may still reduce the PROM. Excessive PROM is common in neurologically impaired patients particularly related to hypotonia, e.g. subluxation of the shoulder. Of course motor control does not have any influence in this case.

ACCESSORY MOVEMENT

The passive accessory range of movement is vital for FROM to be achieved in all joints. In the spinal joints this is termed a 'passive accessory intervertebral movement' (PAIVM).

WHY DO I NEED TO ASSESS RANGE OF MOVEMENT?

A dysfunction of the neural or musculoskeletal systems may lead to joint hypermobility (excessive movement) or hypomobility (reduced movement) either of which may conclude in soft tissue damage, pain and loss of function. Assessment of ROM allows the therapist to identify a potential limitation to functional ability and when combining the findings of AROM and PROM allows the therapist to begin hypothesizing the structures that may be implicated (differential diagnosis).

HOW DO I ASSESS RANGE OF MOVEMENT?

AROM

AROM should be assessed before the PROM is explored.

Patient

The patient's position will alter depending upon the joint being tested because where possible, the position must allow for FROM. For example, full ROM of hip flexion (hip extension to hip flexion) is only possible in standing. In circumstances where this is not practical, such as an immobile patient, the movement will need to be assessed in two halves.

Therapist

The therapist will already have observed the patient's general AROM during the performance of functional activities (S3.18). However, as function involves the combined movement of many joints, a more specific assessment of the individual segments involved *may* be required. Assessment of all the cardinal planes of movement should be considered although clinical judgement should be used as to whether it is necessary to assess every joint and every direction. For example, at the hip the cardinal planes are flexion, extension, abduction, adduction and medial/lateral rotation.

Clinical hints and tips

Based on the subjective assessment and functional objective assessment the therapist needs to use clinical judgement as to whether it is it necessary to assess every joint and every direction.

Limb testing

1. Stand-by assistance or a plinth alongside the patient may be necessary during assessment of the lower limb.
2. The test should be carried out one limb at a time (the unaffected limb first if this is relevant) and measurements taken using a universal goniometer.
3. Choose the appropriate size goniometer for the joint being measured.

4. Demonstrate the movement to ensure the movement is performed correctly.
5. Position the patient to allow FROM.
6. In the start position, place the axis of the goniometer (centre of protractor) over the joint (Fig. 28.1).
7. Line up the stationary arm of the goniometer with a proximal bony landmark that *will not move* during the limb movement (Fig. 28.1).
8. Line up the moveable arm with a bony landmark on the limb that will be moving (Fig. 28.1).
9. Ask the patient to perform the limb movement.
10. At the limit of the patient's ROM, move the moveable arm to line up with the original bony landmark and take the reading (Fig. 28.2).
11. Be sure to read the correct scale from the protractor.
12. The therapist may choose to carry out a *repeated movement* if the test range is reduced. This may elicit a change in the AROM, an increase as they warm up or a decrease as they fatigue.

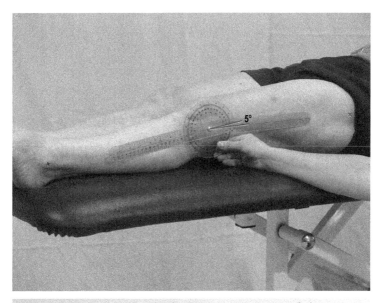

Figure 28.1 Measuring limb ROM: Correct use of the universal goniometer in the start position.

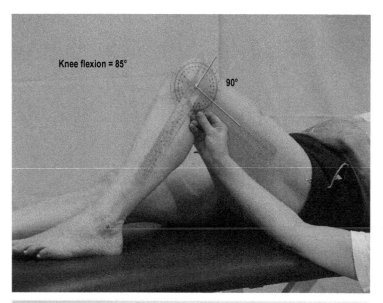

Figure 28.2 Measuring limb ROM: Correct use of the universal goniometer in finish position.

Spinal joint testing   Active physiological movements of the spine involve composite movement of each individual vertebral joint and therefore measurement using a goniometer is not possible. Active spinal movements are therefore measured globally using a tape measure.

1. The patient starts in neutral standing.
2. Make three marks (Fig. 28.3):
   • A horizontal line level with the posterior superior iliac spines
   • 5 cm above this level
   • 10 cm above this level.
3. Ask the patient to move to the finish position (e.g. spinal flexion).
4. At the finish position, re-measure the distances from the posterior superior iliac spine/s (PSIS) level and record (Fig. 28.4).
5. The same procedure can be repeated for extension and side flexion.

Note: Spinal measurements can also be taken from the tip of the third finger to the floor.

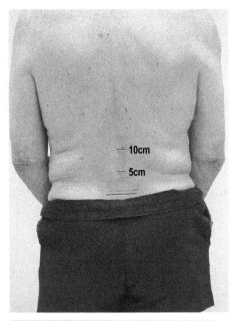

Figure 28.3 Measuring spinal joint ROM: start position.

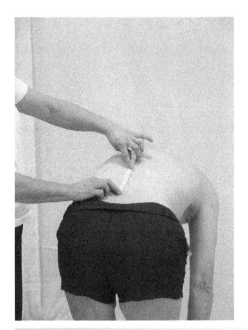

Figure 28.4 Measuring spinal joint ROM: finish position.

Does the patient achieve full active range of movement? This requires the therapist to know the normal values for full AROM of all joints.

Is the AROM excessive or reduced from normal limits?

Is the movement pattern normal? Gross movement patterns may indicate spasticity (S3.21).

Is there any evidence of pain behaviour prior to, during or after the movement? Nociceptive pain may present as avoidance in all or part of the range, facial grimace or verbalization of pain. Neurogenic pain may show no particular link to movement (S3.29).

Are there any compensatory movements used to achieve the range of movement? Compensatory activity may be used in circumstances where the usual muscle/s is/are unable to complete the task (hypotonia, hypertonia, weakness) or the range of the joint is altered (soft tissue adaptation).

PROM

Patient

The patient's position will alter depending upon the joint being tested as where possible, the position must allow for FROM.

Therapist

Spinal joint testing   If a restriction of spinal joint movement is suspected, the therapist should explore the region further using passive physiological intervertebral movements (PPIVMs) and passive accessory intervertebral movements (PAIVMs). These assessment techniques are not covered in this text.

Limb testing   Assessment of all the cardinal planes of movement should be considered, although clinical judgement should be used as to whether it is necessary to assess every joint and every direction. Carrying out PROM is identified as a high-risk manual handling task and therefore consideration of the environment/bed height is essential.

1. The therapist should explain that the movement is to be performed entirely by the therapist.
2. Hold the limb firmly and confidently to allow the patient to relax fully.
3. The therapist should move each segment through the full available ROM.
4. Once the therapist considers they have reached the limit of the patient's ROM, a measurement should be taken accurately and objectively using a universal goniometer. However, more

experienced therapists do use visual estimation. Instructions for the correct use of a goniometer are as for AROM.

Can the therapist achieve full passive range of movement? This requires the therapist to know the normal values for full PROM for all joints.

Is the range of PROM different to that of the AROM? Yes. See analysis section.

Is there any evidence of pain behaviour prior to, during or after the movement? Nociceptive pain may present with guarding/muscle spasm during the testing of PROM. Neurogenic pain may show no particular link to movement (S3.29).

End feel If a *reduced* PROM is identified using passive physiological movements and the patient's pain symptoms are not severe, the therapist may continue to investigate the end feel of the joint so that the structures limiting the ROM can be differentiated during analysis.

1. At the end of the available range the therapist should apply overpressure to the joint in the same direction as the test movement.
2. This additional force must be applied slowly, smoothly and accurately.
3. The therapist should compare the end feel with what they understand to be the normal end feel for that joint. The normal end feels are different according to the structures limiting the joint (Magee 2006).
   a. Soft end feel: Related to soft tissue apposition (e.g. knee flexion)
   b. Hard end feel: Related to bone to bone (e.g. elbow extension)
   c. Firm/springy end feel: Related to tissue stretch (e.g. ankle dorsiflexion)
   d. Capsular restriction (e.g. in shoulder and hip lateral rotation).

Note: Hypertonia may restrict the AROM well before the end of PROM. If possible the therapist still needs to investigate the end feel beyond the hypertonic restriction to explore the existence of any soft tissue adaptation.

What is the end feel of the joint at the end of its range? The resistance is considered abnormal if the normal end feel is not present or the resistance is felt too early in the normal range (Petty 2006).

RECORDING

The recording of this data could be extensive. It may therefore be wise to note the findings in a list or table form.

ANALYSIS

The therapist's analysis of ROM will inform other areas of the objective assessment. For example, reduced AROM of the ankle dorsiflexors may explain abnormal gait and poor balance. The aim of this assessment tool is to establish the patient's ROM and to begin hypothesizing about any possible limiting factors. In the case of a reduced ROM, this can be achieved by comparing the findings from both AROM and PROM assessments. For example, if PROM is greater than AROM then a deficit of muscle contraction should be suspected. This could be caused by muscle weakness, hypotonia, hypertonia or sensory loss. However, if both PROM and AROM are reduced, the limit is more likely to be linked with a soft tissue adaptation. Note: Pain could be a causal factor in both these scenarios and needs further investigation (S3.29).

OUTCOME MEASURES

RESEARCH
- Silicon COACH
- VICON.

CLINICAL
- Goniometry
- Silicon COACH.

REFERENCES AND FURTHER READING
Fox J, Day R: *A physiotherapist's guide to clinical measurement*, Edinburgh, 2009, Churchill Livingstone/Elsevier.

Magee DJ: *Orthopaedic physical assessment*, ed 4, Canada, 2006, Elsevier Sciences.

Petty NJ: *Neuromusculoskeletal examination and assessment: a handbook for therapists*, Edinburgh, 2006, Churchill Livingstone.

Pain

WHAT IS PAIN?

'an unpleasant sensory and emotional experience associated with actual or potential tissue damage, or described in terms of such damage'
(International Association for the Study of Pain (IASP) 2007)

Pain is highly complex with many interactive dimensions, including physiological, sensory, affective, cognitive, behavioural and psychosocial. The evidence base related to pain is often confusing for the novice therapist because of the different terminology used in different areas of speciality and a lack of clarification between types of pain, the physiological processes involved and the signs and symptoms presented. This section will attempt to summarize the issues surrounding pain, related to the neurologically impaired patient. For more in depth reading, the therapist is referred to the International Association for the Study of Pain (IASP) website (www.iasp-pain.org).

TYPES OF PAIN

There are three main types of pain experienced by neurologically impaired patients, with patients often presenting with more than one type.

- Nociceptive (including dystonia S3.18)
- Psychogenic
- Neuropathic.

Nociceptive

This type of pain is physiological and arises as a consequence of the *activation of nociceptors* (pain receptors) following a chemical, thermal or mechanical event. The activation of primary nociceptive afferents by actual or potentially tissue-damaging stimuli is then processed within the nociceptive system (Treede et al. 2008). This type of pain may involve the musculoskeletal system but can also be from a visceral origin. It is important to note that not all nociceptive activation is perceived by the individual as 'pain'. The perception of an unpleasant experience (pain) is highly subjective. *Dystonic pain* is associated with abnormal sustained muscle contraction (S3.18), which mediates the activation of nociceptive afferents in the muscles.

Psychogenic

This is pain that is caused, increased, or prolonged by cognitive, emotional, or behavioural factors. The IASP (2007) describe psychogenic pain as:

> 'reported pain in the absence of tissue damage or any likely pathophysiological cause. There is usually no way to distinguish their experience from that due to tissue damage if we take the subjective report. If they regard their experience as pain and if they report it in the same ways as pain caused by tissue damage, it should be accepted as pain'.

Neuropathic

This type of pain arises by activity generated within the nociceptive system *without adequate stimulation of its peripheral sensory endings (nociceptors)* and is caused by a primary lesion or dysfunction in the nervous system (IASP 2007). Some authors have further narrowed the dysfunction to a lesion of the somatosensory system (Treede et al. 2008). This includes the afferent neuron, the ascending and descending pathways, medulla, thalamus, or cerebral cortex. Therefore, neuropathic pain is sub-divided in relation to the anatomical site of the lesion (Dworkin et al. 2003).

Peripheral neuropathic pain This involves pain as a result of damage to the peripheral nervous system (PNS).

Central neuropathic pain This involves pain associated with central nervous system (CNS) damage.

PHYSIOLOGY OF PAIN

The experience of pain has a protective role which warns us of imminent or actual tissue damage and elicits responses, via signals within the nervous system, which keep such damage to a minimum. This brings about temporary pain hypersensitivity in the inflamed and adjacent tissue (peripheral sensitization). This process assists healing as contact and movement will be avoided. However, persistent pain offers no benefits and can be extremely debilitating. This maladaptive pain often occurs following damage to the peripheral nerve, the spinal cord or the CNS and is termed neuropathic pain (Woolfe and Mannion 1999). Figure 29.1 shows a simple flowchart outlining the normal pain pathway and the processes involved in pathological pain.

SYMPTOMS ASSOCIATED WITH PAIN

Nociceptive pain and peripheral neuropathic pain

The symptoms associated with these types of pain are comprehensively covered in many basic physiology texts. More detailed guidance can be sought from a range of musculoskeletal texts in relation to assessment and treatment.

Central neuropathic pain (CNP)

Unfortunately there are no uniform predictable signs with regard to the clinical presentation of CNP and the descriptions often vary greatly between patients. As a result it is often diagnosed through exclusion of any other source.

The symptoms of CNP occur as a result of CNS damage particularly to the somatosensory system which may lead to disinhibition and central sensitization (Fig. 29.1). With the pain pathway now inappropriately active, activity dependent neural plastic changes occur at the synapses within the whole pathway and may lead to an increase in the cortical representation (sensory homunculus) of the painful part. The timescales within which

Mechanisms of pain	Pain pathway

NOCICEPTIVE PAIN

1. Peripheral sensitization

Primary hyperalgesia – Increased sensitivity of the nociceptors (pain receptors) adjacent to the damaged area in response to chemicals released during the healing process. This is a normal safety mechanism to avoid further damage. *Secondary hyperalgesia* – This involves sensitization of nociceptors some distance from the initial damage possibly innervated by branches of the neurons affected by primary hyperalgesia. This occurs some time later, but no timeframe is given as absolute (Kandel et al 2000).

NEUROPATHIC PAIN
PERIPHERAL OR CENTRAL

1. Prolonged peripheral sensitization

2. Central sensitization occurs some time later because of the increased barrage of pain information entering the dorsal horn. As a result, the pain afferents in laminar II may sprout and the existing synapses become more efficient (neuroplasticity). The outcome being that the pain pathway is strengthened and therefore requires less stimulation to produce the same experience of pain (Loeser and Treede 2008). Laminar III and IV transmitting tactile signals lie adjacent to the pain tracts; consequently they may be similarly affected by these neuroplastic adaptations. Ultimately an increased sensitivity of these tactile pathways can lead to tactile sensations being perceived abnormally or as pain.

3. Disinhibition or loss of descending inhibition – Damage to the central nervous system involving the descending pain tract, somatosensory cortex, mid-brain (PAG) or spinal cord may result in a loss of inhibitory modulation by PAG at the dorsal horn. Consequently there will be an inappropriately heightened perception of pain which may not reflect the pain stimulus.

Stimulation of nociceptors by chemical, thermal or mechanical event
Potential tissue damage

Primary nociceptive afferents activated (A delta and c fibres) which transmit pain to the dorsal horn of the spinal cord. Synapse primarily in laminar I, II, V–VII.

Pain ascends in the spinothalamic, spinoreticular and the spinomesencephalic tracts to various regions of the mid-brain. Pain is modulated by peri aqueductal grey (PAG) (mid-brain). PAG decides on action depending on the strength of the stimulus.

PAG can directly block a non-significant stimulus from being passed on to higher centres.

If the stimulus is significant PAG will pass the pain information to the thalamus where a crude pain is perceived and on to the somatosensory cortex in parietal lobe where pain can be localized.

If the stimulus is significant, PAG can send a signal back down to the dorsal horn in the spinal cord to release endorphins and encephalins. These neurotransmitters activate an inhibitory interneuron within the dorsal horn that **reduces the transmission of incoming pain** information so that perception of pain is reduced.

Figure 29.1 Pathophysiology of pain.

these neural changes take place and in which the symptoms develop is not clear with different studies stating from 1 month to 5–6 years.

The symptoms produced as a result of disinhibition and central sensitization include:

Hyperalgesia   This is an increased sensitivity to pain.

Allodynia   This is pain perceived following a non-noxious stimulus which does not normally provoke pain (e.g. touch, heat or non-noxious cold). This is common (90%) in central neuropathic pain (Widar et al. 2002).

Hyperpathia   This is an unpleasant, prolonged post-stimulus reaction.

Dysaesthesia   This is an unpleasant abnormal sensation. For example, burning, wetness, itching, electric shock, pins and needles. This is common in CNP (80%) (Attal et al. 2008).

Paraesthesia   This is an abnormal but not unpleasant sensation.

Behaviour of CNP symptoms   The symptoms of CNP may be *spontaneous* when they present from no apparent source, *evoked* as an over-reaction to a wide variety of stimuli, *persistent* (consistent/permanent) or *paroxysmal* (temporary).

Distribution of neuropathic pain   *Peripheral neuropathic pain*: In PNS lesions the pain distribution will conform to the cutaneous innervation of the peripheral nerve, the branches of the brachial or lumbar plexus, or spinal roots (dermatomes).

Central neuropathic pain: In CNS lesions the pain distribution will conform to the topographical representation of the brain area that has been injured by the lesion (i.e. the sensory homunculus). However, as central sensitization is one of the mechanisms that contributes to neuropathic pain, abnormal expansions of the sensory map should be expected.

Central neuropathic pain in neurologically impaired patients

Although neurological conditions result from very different pathophysiology, the pathological processes involved can still be identified as causal in producing CNP. For example, demyelination in MS, compromised circulation in CVA and disruption of spinal cord transmission in SCI can all involve damage to the somatosensory system and therefore produce CNP.

Recent studies have also highlighted a further process that may contribute to CNP which involves the action of glial cells following a CNS lesion. In SCI and MS, inflammatory changes initiated in response to cell damage promote the release of inflammatory mediators and growth hormones by glial cells. If these chemical mediators affect the pain pathway, central sensitization may be enhanced (Svendsen et al. 2005). Although this has not been reported in CVA, it is likely that a similar mechanism takes place following the initial lesion and the resultant inflammatory response.

In PD the mechanism of CNP may be different. In healthy individuals the basal ganglia (S2.11) is now thought to play a significant role in the integration of sensory information and hence the modulation of pain (Juri et al. 2009). In PD the pathophysiology of pain has been linked to a disruption of the basal ganglia's (striatum) ability to filter the vast amounts of sensory information in order to select an appropriate movement programme. This filtering is normally facilitated by the inhibitory dopaminergic neurons, however as the latter undergoes neurodegeneration in PD its effect is reduced. This may explain why pain may be relieved when in an 'on' period (i.e. taking L-Dopa).

WHY DO I NEED TO ASSESS PAIN?

While the available knowledge about pain, its physiology and pathophysiology has increased enormously over the last 20 years, it appears to have been largely ignored in respect to patients with neurological deficits. Pain in this population requires recognition as it has been shown to impact significantly on the patient's quality of life and on the rehabilitative process (Henon 2006).

The incidence of pain in neurologically impaired patients is high, with reports of up to 74% in CVA and SCI; 50–85% in MS and between 40% and 75% in PD. A further breakdown of the different types of pain presented in these conditions can be seen in Tables 29.1–29.3

HOW DO I ASSESS PAIN?

Pain in the neurologically impaired patient is often complex and should be assessed thoroughly. The following offers a brief overview of the main considerations when assessing pain. Initially the therapist should try to establish the type of pain experienced by the patient, remembering that this population often have pain of more than one type.

Table 29.1 Incidence of different types of pain in cerebrovascular accident

Nociceptive pain	5–84%
Shoulder pain	30–40%
Chronic pain	11–55%
Central neuropathic pain	2–35%
Central post-stroke pain	8–46%

Widar et al. 2002; Jönsson et al. 2006; Lindgren et al. 2007; Kong and Woon 2004; Appelros 2006; Kumar and Soni 2009.

Table 29.2 Incidence of different types of pain in Parkinson's disease

Nociceptive pain	40–70%
Non-dystonic	37.8%
Dystonic	6.7–40%
Peripheral neuropathic pain	10%
Central neuropathic pain	4.5–30%

DeFazio and Tinazzi 2009; Beiske et al. 2009; Djaldetti et al. 2004.

Table 29.3 Incidence of different types of pain in multiple sclerosis

Nociceptive pain	21% (1% related to spasticity)
Peripheral neuropathic pain	1%
Central neuropathic pain	27.5% (87% in LL: 31% in UL)
Abnormal response to pain and temperature	98%

Osterberg et al. 2005.

SUBJECTIVE ASSESSMENT

Enquiry related to the following is required:

Onset of pain

Question about the time of onset and any causal event linked to onset.

Area of pain

Identify a location of pain from the patient. This will help to start focusing in on certain structures. However, referred pain away from the origin of the pain means that this information cannot be relied upon completely. If pain reports are diffuse and widespread, the therapist may start to suspect central neuropathic or psychogenic pain.

Behaviour of the symptoms

This questioning should include the pattern of pain in terms of the 24-hour day and any factors that increase or decrease their symptoms (known as aggravating and easing factors). The acronym SIN is often used to represent other information that should be sought:

Severity of the pain (intensity). See visual analogue scale below.
Irritability of the pain, how long does it take for pain to reduce to previous level after a stimulus is removed?
Nature of the pain, a description of the symptoms of pain experienced.

Does the patient describe their pain using adjectives that are typically linked with physiological mechanisms? For example, a dull ache which is difficult to localize (muscle, ligament, joint capsule pain); morning pain that improves with activity (chronic inflammation/oedema); bizarre descriptions of pins and needles; wetness (central neuropathic pain); a sharp or burning pain or a line of pain (peripheral neuropathic pain).

Does the patient report a pattern of pain behaviour? The description of a typical pattern of pain behaviour may help identify a nociceptive origin. No pattern of pain behaviour may indicate a central neuropathic or psychogenic origin.

Does the patient report an irritable condition? The therapist will need to take care during the assessment and treatment not to aggravate their symptoms.

Visual analogue scale (VAS)

The VAS allows the therapist to assess the patient's perception of their pain in terms of intensity/severity. This test can be carried out on initial assessment and during follow-up treatments to monitor the level of pain in relation to the effectiveness of interventions.

Patient Patient should be seated comfortably at a table.
Therapist
1. The therapist draws a horizontal line on a piece of paper 10 cm long. The left hand end indicates a 0 score (no pain) and the right hand end a 10 score (the worst pain imaginable) (Fig. 29.2).

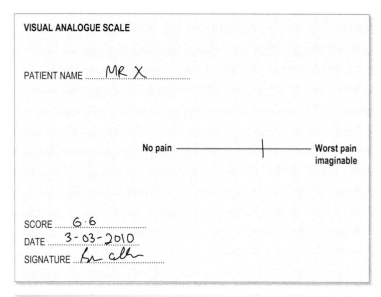

Figure 29.2 Visual analogue scale.

2. The patient is requested to rate their *perceived pain* intensity *at that moment in time* by making *one* mark on the line between the two extreme scores.
3. The therapist can then measure along the line from 0 to the point where the patient placed their mark. This value can be used as a quantitative marker for future evaluation.

The Neuropathic Pain Symptom Inventory (NPSI)

The Neuropathic Pain Symptom Inventory (NPSI) (Bouhassira et al. 2004) presents a broad overview of central neuropathic pain symptoms and may be useful to use as a reference source to assist the novice practitioner in identifying the signs of central neuropathic pain from the subjective assessment. Although it is often possible to diagnose neuropathic pain on the basis of history, a clinical examination is also essential (Treede et al. 2008).

OBJECTIVE ASSESSMENT

Observation

As the perception of pain is subjective, the therapist should also look for other signs and behaviours which may indicate pain. This process can be ongoing from the time the patient enters the department until the time they leave:

a. Muscle spasm guarding an area
b. Facial grimacing and either increased or decreased vocalizations during movement
c. Poor posture
d. Decreased range or altered patterns of movement
e. Altered muscle tone (S3.21)
f. Dystonia (S3.18)
g. Altered appetite and weight
h. Anxious and stressed. These factors may exacerbate pain
i. Fatigue/exhaustion. This may reflect a lack of sleep due to pain
j. Low mood and poor concentration. Depression may also exacerbate pain
k. Socially withdrawn.

Distribution of pain and other sensations

Assessment of:

- Pin prick testing (S3.23)
- Temperature testing (S3.23)
- Light touch testing (S3.23).

Does the patient exhibit an increased sensitivity to pain? This is hyperalgesia.

Does the patient exhibit a decreased sensitivity to pain? This is hypoalgesia.

Does the patient exhibit an abnormal pain response to a non-noxious stimulus? This is allodynia.

Does the patient report an unpleasant abnormal sensation? (e.g. burning, wetness, itching, electric shock, pins and needles). This is dysaesthesia.

Does the pattern of pain conform to the specific distribution of dermatomes or peripheral nerves? Yes. This is peripheral neuropathic pain. If not it is likely to reflect central neuropathic pain.

DIFFERENTIAL DIAGNOSIS OF NOCICEPTIVE PAIN

At this stage the therapist may have made a reasoned decision as to the type of pain (nociceptive, peripheral or central neuropathic) being experienced by the patient.

If the patient's pain is considered to be of nociceptive origin, a comparison of the findings from AROM (S3.23) and PROM (S3.23) and special clinical tests will allow the therapist to differentiate the structures implicated. In each case, the therapist is evaluating the reproduction of the patient's pain in order to identify the source. Further comprehensive detail guiding differential diagnosis can be found from a range of musculoskeletal based texts.

Caution
Although reproducing the patient's pain during the assessment is
necessary, be careful not to aggravate the intensity of the pain.

RECORDING

A separate section in your subjective write up should be headed
'Pain', with sub-headings as suggested in the above text. For the
objective findings, a body chart showing the distribution of pain
is a clear and easy way to present the information (Fig. 29.3). Use
different symbols to highlight the various symptoms. The visual
analogue scale (Fig. 29.2) should be included and the numeric
result recorded in your notes.

Example Patient diagnosed with CVA affecting the right parietal
lobe (medially).

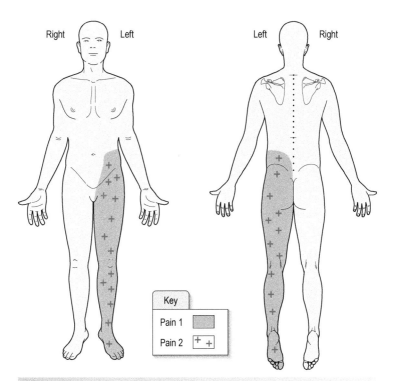

Figure 29.3 Example of a body chart recording (pain).

Onset of pain was 6/52 (6 weeks) post-CVA. Pain 1 is initiated by light touch and pain 2 relates to increased sensitivity to pin prick testing. Figure 29.3 shows the distribution of pain 1 and 2. There appears to be no discernible pattern to the pain behaviour. Pain is spontaneous and unaffected by movement or posture.

ANALYSIS

Based upon the patient's diagnosis and findings from the pain assessment the therapist should be able to use clinical reasoning skills to identify the type of pain, discriminating between nociceptive or neuropathic origin. This is vital, as understanding the pathological processes involved will facilitate more effective and focused treatment.

As central neuropathic pain is traditionally treated with medication, a referral to the medical team is indicated if the symptoms are not already being managed. Cognitive/behavioural therapy and mirror therapy are also options which the therapist may consider.

For nociceptive pain, the therapist should also aim to identify the structure responsible for the nociceptive activation in order to focus treatment appropriately. This requires a reasoning process involving knowledge of anatomy, the possible mechanisms of injury related to different structures and the physiological processes involved in healing. For further guidance, the reader is referred to Grieve (2006). Remember that the source of pain may also be visceral in nature.

In the example above, the patient presents with hyperalgesia and allodynia involving the left lower limb. As no pattern of pain behaviour is evident and the location reflects the area of somatosensory cortex damage, this is assumed to be central neuropathic pain.

OUTCOME MEASURES

RESEARCH
- Algometry
- Pain matcher.

CLINICAL
- Visual analogue scale
- McGill–Melzack pain questionnaire
- Neuropathic Pain Symptom Inventory.

REFERENCES AND FURTHER READING

Appelros P: Prevalence and predictors of pain and fatigue after stroke: a population-based study, *International Journal of Rehabilitation Research* 29:329–333, 2006.

Attal N, Fermanian C, Fermanian J, et al: Neuropathic pain: are there distinct subtypes depending on the aetiology or anatomical lesion? *Pain* 138:343–353, 2008.

Beiske AG, Loge JH, Ronningen A, et al: Pain in Parkinson's disease: the hidden epidemic, *Pain* 141:173–177, 2009.

Bouhassira D, Attal N, Fermanian J, et al: Development and validation of the neuropathic pain symptom inventory, *Pain* 108:248–257, 2004.

Day R, Fox J, Paul-Taylor G: *Neuro-musculoskeletal clinical tests: a clinician's guide.* Edinburgh, 2009, Churchill Livingstone/Elsevier.

DeFazio G, Tinazzi M: Central pain and Parkinson's disease, *Archives of Neurology* 66:282–283, 2009.

Djaldetti R, Shifrin A, Rogowski Z, et al: Quantitative measurement of pain sensation in patients with Parkinson's disease, *Neurology* 62:2171–2175, 2004.

Dworkin RH, Backonja M, Rowbotham MC, et al: Advances in neuropathic pain: diagnosis mechanisms and treatment recommendations, *Archives of Neurology* 60:1524–1534, 2003.

Ehde DM, Gibbons LE, Chwastiak L, et al. Chronic pain in a large community sample of persons with multiple sclerosis, *Multiple Sclerosis* 9:605–611, 2003.

Finnerup NB: A review of central neuropathic pain states, *Current Opinion in Anaesthesiology* 21:586–589, 2008.

Grieve DJ: *Orthopaedic physical assessment*, ed 4. Canada, 2006, Saunders Elsevier.

Henon H: Pain after stroke: a neglected issue, *Journal of Neurology Neurosurgery and Psychiatry* 77:569, 2006.

IASP, International Association for the Study of Pain: wwwiasp-painorg/AM/Templatecfm?Section=Pain_DefinitionsandTemplate=/CM/HTMLDisplaycfmandContentID=1728, 2007.

Jönsson AC, Lindgren I, Hallstrom B et al: Prevalence and intensity of pain after stroke: a population based study focusing on patients' perspectives, *Journal of Neurology, Neurosurgery and Psychiatry* 77:590–595, 2006.

Juri C, Rodriguez-Oroz M, Obeso JA: The pathophysiological basis of sensory disturbances in Parkinson's disease, *Journal of Neurologic Science* 289:60–65, 2009.

Kandel ER, Schwartz JH, Jessell TM: *Principles of neural science*, ed 4. New York, 2000, McGraw-Hill.

Kong KH, Woon VC, Yang SY: Prevalence of chronic pain and its impact on health-related quality of life in stroke survivors, *Archives of Physical Medicine and Rehabilitation* 85: 35–40, 2004.

Kumar G, Soni CR: Central post-stroke pain: Current evidence, *Journal of Neurologic Science* 284:10–17, 2009.

Lindgren I, Jönsson AC, Norrving B et al: Shoulder pain after stroke: a prospective population-based study, *Stroke* 38:343–348, 2007.

Loeser JD, Treede RD: The Kyoto protocol of IASP basic pain terminology, *Pain* 137:473–477, 2008.

Osterberg A, Boivie J, Thuomas K-A: Central pain in multiple sclerosis: prevalence and clinical characteristics, *European Journal of Pain* 9:531–542, 2005.

Svendsen KB, Jensen TS, Hansen HJ, et al: Sensory function and quality of life in patients with multiple sclerosis and pain, *Pain* 114:473–481, 2005.

Treede RD, Jensen TS, Campbell JN, et al: Neuropathic pain: redefinition and a grading system for clinical and research purposes, *Neurology* 7018:1630–1635, 2008.

Widar M, Samuelsson L, Karlsson-Tivenius S, et al: Long-term pain conditions after a stroke, *Journal of Rehabilitation Medicine* 34:165–170, 2002.

Woolfe CJ, Mannion RJ: Neuropathic pain: aetiology, symptoms, mechanisms and management, *The Lancet* 353:1959–1964, 1999.

Strength

WHAT IS MUSCLE STRENGTH?

Normal muscle strength is defined as the maximum force a muscle can generate in a specified movement pattern (Knuttgen and Kraemer 1987). Muscle weakness being interpreted as the inability to generate sufficient force to complete a task in a given context. In other words the muscle itself may be able to recruit sufficient force under certain circumstances but not in others when it will present as weak. As well as the context and the task itself, force production in a muscle is influenced by many factors associated with the anatomy and physiology of the muscle and the nervous system controlling it:

- *Motor unit* (an alpha motor neuron and the muscle fibres supplied by it)
  - Number recruited. The greater the number, the greater the force
  - Order of recruitment. To produce a smooth coordinated muscle contraction, small motor units are recruited before

larger units. This is termed the size principle or Henneman principle

- Size of motor unit. This relates to muscle fibre type, with larger motor units comprised of type IIx (fast glycolytic) fibres and smaller units made up of type I (slow oxidative) fibres
- Frequency of the firing rate. An increased frequency of muscle action potentials to the neuromuscular junction results in summation (S2.6) of the signals.

Generally, greater force is generated with an increased number and size of motor units and at an increased rate of firing.

- *Psychological factors* such as motivation and mood also affect force production
- *Cross-sectional area*: The greater the cross-sectional area of the muscle, the greater the number of muscle fibres, motor units and ultimately sarcomeres that can be recruited in *parallel* and therefore the greater the force generated. Compare the force produced when pulling a car using a single rope with the force generated when 10 ropes are used (in parallel). However, the cross-sectional area includes both contractile and non-contractile tissue, the latter of which does not contribute to force production.
- *Neural control*: The force production of a given muscle is governed by the task requirements in terms of:
  - Timing
  - Pattern
  - Level of force.

For a learned movement task these factors are integrated into the stored movement plan of the task which then provides feed forward prediction of the force requirements. However, the force production is also modified by ongoing sensory input from the periphery.

- Other factors
  - The length tension relationship within the muscle relates to the potential for actin and myosin cross-bridge formation. Working in middle range of the muscle provides the optimum number of available cross-bridges and hence the greatest force production
  - The anatomical alignment of muscle fibre within an individual muscle also influences force production (Palastanga et al. 2006)
  - The type of muscle work, concentric eccentric or isometric.

MUSCLE WEAKNESS

Muscle weakness may occur as a result of:

- Partial or complete lesion of a peripheral nerve
- Injury to the musculoskeletal system resulting in inflammation, oedema and pain
- Pain which may cause the inhibition of muscle contraction (S3.29)
- A change in role of a muscle imposed by damage to the musculoskeletal or nervous systems may lead to a change in muscle fibre type
- Altered neural control affecting the recruitment of motor units
- Decreased use of the muscle which causes:
  - A change in muscle length, becoming lengthened or shortened
  - Muscle atrophy, whereby muscle proteins (actin and myosin myofilaments) are lost. Locally there is a loss of sarcomeres in the muscle fibre and globally a reduction in muscle mass (Ryan et al. 2002) and cross-sectional area.

Weakness in neurological conditions   Disorders affecting the peripheral nervous system such as Guillain–Barré syndrome and motor neuron disease often present with weakness as a primary symptom. Damage to the alpha motor neurons interferes with the nerve conduction, which ultimately means that insufficient motor units are recruited and muscle weakness presents. Secondary to this, further weakness may occur as a result of disuse, leading to a loss of sarcomeres and therefore muscle mass (atrophy) (Ryan et al. 2002). Following damage to the peripheral nervous system, motor units can be re-innervated via regeneration of the damaged neuron. However, if the nerve lesion is a long distance from a completely denervated motor unit it may be re-innervated as a result of axonal sprouting from adjacent alpha motor neurons. If this sprouting is heterotypic (not from the same muscle fibre type) the patient may present with dysfunctional incoordinated movement (Lieber 2002). This is a consequence of a disruption in the order of recruitment of motor units (the size principle). The recruitment of small units (type I) followed by the larger units (type IIx) ensures that the force of contraction is built up slowly and smoothly. However, if sprouting occurs from a neuron innervating a type I motor unit to re-innervate a type IIx motor unit the outcome will be large increases in force production too early in the sequence of recruitment and hence an incoordinated movement.

In disorders of the central nervous system (CNS) such as cerebrovascular accident (CVA), Parkinson's disease and multiple sclerosis, the mechanism underlying muscle weakness is a consequence of damage to higher centres or the pathways involved in motor control. This results in altered signalling down the descending tracts to the alpha motor neuron pool in the spinal cord, the outcome of which is a dysfunction in the timing or pattern of motor unit recruitment or the number of units being recruited. However, ultimately these factors may lead to insufficient or inappropriate recruitment of motor units in a given context and consequently insufficient force to overcome the resistance of the task, or weakness (paresis). Over time, the reduced force production will also be contributed to by a loss of sarcomeres and therefore muscle mass (atrophy) as a consequence of disuse (Ryan et al. 2002). This secondary onset muscle weakness is a common symptom in neurologically impaired patients and may present in any circumstance which leads to movement dysfunction and disuse, e.g. motor impairments but also sensory impairment (S3.23) and cognitive/perceptual deficits (S3.33).

In CNS lesions, muscle weakness is evident in association with both hypotonia (reduced muscle tone) and hypertonia (increased muscle tone; S3.21). The relationship between these concepts is complex but it appears likely that both altered tone states are contributory factors that negatively influence force production (weakness). The pathophysiology which defines alterations in muscle tone also leads to a dysfunction in the timing or pattern of motor unit recruitment or the number of units able to be recruited. Therefore, muscle weakness during movement may be apparent. In terms of assessment a comparison of the conceptual definitions of tone and weakness gives the therapist a simplified tool by which to differentiate. Muscle tone is defined as the resistance to passive movement, representing the background level of tension or stiffness in a muscle (Moore and Kowalske 2000). Therefore it should be assessed in a muscle at rest. Muscle weakness on the other hand is defined as the inability to generate sufficient force to overcome the resistance of a task and therefore by definition should be assessed during movement activities.

WHY DO I NEED TO ASSESS MUSCLE STRENGTH?

Normal muscle strength is required to function in our activities of daily living. Any weakness may lead to ineffective unsuccessful movement with the potential for creating excessive stresses on soft tissue structures which may lead to pain and movement avoidance. By assessing general and/or individual muscle strength, the therapist will be able to focus a strengthening regime to assist the patient in achieving their full potential. However, while focusing upon specific weakened muscles it is also vital to simultaneously re-educate and integrate the strengthened muscles back into functional activities.

In CVA, muscle weakness has been shown to be the major contributor to limits in functional ability (Chae et al. 2002; Kim and Eng 2003; Mercier and Bourbonnais 2004). However, it is still widely believed that resistance strength training increases muscle tone and is therefore avoided in patients with central nervous disorders. However, this belief appears unwarranted when considering the evidence to the contrary. Several studies have now reported significant gains in strength without detrimental increases in spasticity in CVA (Sharp and Brouwer 1997; Brown and Kautz 1998; Badics et al. 2002; Sterr and Freivogel 2004; Morris et al. 2004; Ada et al. 2006) and multiple sclerosis (Taylor et al. 2006). The research also indicates that the increases in strength through resistance training are transferred into some functional improvement in CVA (Yang et al. 2006; Ada et al. 2006; Bale and Strand 2008) and multiple sclerosis (Taylor et al. 2006).

HOW DO I ASSESS MUSCLE STRENGTH?

Strength measures utilized by the therapist may involve isometric (static), isokinetic/isotonic (dynamic – concentric and eccentric) testing, functional activities or lifting weights (1 repetition maximum). The choice of assessment will be dependent upon the test requirements.

MUSCLE CROSS-SECTIONAL AREA (LIMB GIRTH MEASUREMENT)

As a muscle's size is proportional to its strength, a simple measure of muscle bulk gives the therapist a clue about muscle strength in terms of hypertrophy or atrophy when compared with the other side of the body. However, hand dominance will need to be taken into account. The limitation of this measure is that it also includes the non-contractile elements of the muscle and does not tell the therapist about the level of force production.

Patient The measurement should be carried out on a relaxed muscle and therefore the patient should be well supported in either supine or long sitting during the assessment.
Therapist

1. Mark on the limb 2 or 3 points of reference (Table 30.1, Fig. 30.1) depending upon the size of the limb. A standardized system of taking the measurements will improve repeatability

Table 30.1 Standardized markers for measuring limb girth

Limb girth measurement	Markers for measurement
Limb girth – thigh	15 cm, 20 cm, 25 cm superior to the tibial tuberosity (Fig. 30.1)
Limb girth – calf	5 cm, 10 cm, 15 cm inferiorly to the tibial tuberosity
Limb girth – upper limb (upper arm)	4 cm and 8 cm superiorly from the olecranon process
Limb girth – upper limb (forearm)	4 cm inferiorly from the olecranon process

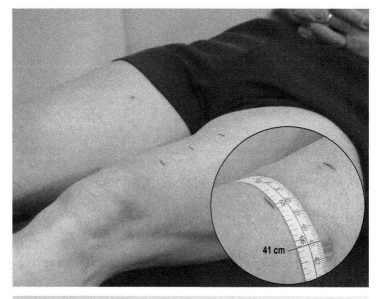

Figure 30.1 Example of limb girth measurement (thigh).

2. Use a tape measure to measure the circumference of the limb at each mark
3. Repeat the measurement 3 times for each mark
4. Calculate the average for each mark
5. Repeat on the other side and compare.

Clinical hints and tips
Consistency. Use the tape measure superiorly to all the marks (Fig. 30.1) or inferiorly. Record the option used for future reference.

MANUAL MUSCLE STRENGTH TESTING
The most commonly used methods are:

- Isometric resisted movement: Used for differential diagnosis to implicate contractile tissue or to test nerve integrity (myotomes).
- Oxford grading (Dyck et al. 2005). This assessment utilizes a measurement scale from 0–5 (Medical Research Council 1976).

The grades are defined as:

0 – No contraction
1 – Flicker or trace of contraction
2 – Full active range of movement with gravity eliminated
3 – Full active range of movement against gravity
4 – Full active range of movement against gravity and against minimal resistance
5 – Full range of movement against gravity and against maximal resistance (normal strength).

Oxford grading (MRC scale)
Patient As the grades are defined in relation to the full active range of movement (ROM) and in relation to gravity, the position of the patient may need to be modified when testing each joint, each direction of movement and each grade. Table 30.2 provides a guide to the patient's position necessary for each test to be completed. The patient needs to be sufficiently undressed to allow the therapist to observe and/or palpate the muscle being assessed. Palpating through clothes is not good practice.

Table 30.2 Guide to the positioning of the patient during the assessment of manual muscle testing for grades 0–5 (MRC scale)

Muscle action	Patient position in relation to grade being tested		
	Grades 0 and 1	Grade 2	Grades 3, 4 and 5
Hip extensors	Prone	Side lying	Prone – lower limb over the edge of plinth to start in full hip flexion
Hip flexors	Supine	Side lying	Supine – lower limb over edge of plinth to start in full hip extension
Hip abductors	Supine	Supine	Side lying or standing[a]
Hip adductors	Supine	Supine	Side lying or standing[a]
Hip lateral rotators	Prone	Supine	Sitting – hips and knees at 90°
Hip medial rotators	Supine	Supine	Sitting – hips and knees at 90°
Knee extensors	Supine	Side lying	Sitting
Knee flexors	Prone	Side lying	Prone or standing
Ankle plantar flexors	Prone	Side lying	Prone or standing
Ankle dorsiflexors	Supine	Side lying	Supine or sitting
Ankle evertors	Supine	Supine	Side lying with foot off the edge of the plinth to start in full ankle inversion
Ankle invertors	Supine	Supine	Side lying with foot off the edge of the plinth to start in full ankle eversion
Shoulder extensors	Prone	Side lying	Sitting or standing[a] Supine – prone
Shoulder flexors	Supine	Side lying	Sitting or standing[a] Supine – prone[a]

[a]Therapist needs to consider using two postures when testing.

Muscle action	Patient position in relation to grade being tested		
	Grades 0 and 1	Grade 2	Grades 3, 4 and 5
Shoulder abductors	Supine	Supine	Standing with shoulder in slight flexion to avoid trunk
Shoulder adductors	Supine	Supine	Standing with shoulder in slight flexion to avoid trunk
Shoulder lateral rotators	Prone	Sitting with elbow 90°	Side lying (top arm)
Shoulder medial rotators	Supine	Sitting with elbow 90°	Side lying trunk at 45° (bottom arm)
Elbow extensors	Prone	Side lying or sitting with shoulder in 90 degrees abduction	Prone or sitting at hand table with shoulder in full extension
Elbow flexors	Supine	Side lying or sitting with shoulder in 90° abduction	Supine or sitting at hand table
Forearm supinators	Supine or sitting	It is difficult to eliminate gravity in full ROM	Grade 3 – it is difficult to complete full ROM against gravity. Supine or sitting at hand table (elbow extended and forearm pronated)
Forearm pronators	Supine or sitting	It is difficult to eliminate gravity in full ROM	Grade 3 – it is difficult to complete full ROM against gravity. Supine or sitting at hand table (elbow extended and forearm supinated)
Wrist extensors	Supine or sitting	Supine or sitting with forearm in mid position	Supine or sitting at hand table (hand off table) with forearm pronated
Wrist flexors	Supine or sitting	Supine or sitting with forearm in mid position	Supine or sitting at hand table (hand off table) with forearm supinated

table continues

Muscle action	Patient position in relation to grade being tested		
	Grades 0 and 1	Grade 2	Grades 3, 4 and 5
Wrist ulnar deviators	Supine or sitting	Supine or sitting with forearm pronated	Supine or sitting at hand table (hand off table) with shoulder medially rotated and forearm pronated
Wrist radial deviators	Supine or sitting	Supine or sitting with forearm pronated	Supine or sitting at hand table (hand off table) with forearm in mid position
Thumb abductors and adductors and finger extensors and flexors (movement in frontal plane)	Supine or sitting	Supine or sitting with forearm in mid position	Supine or sitting at hand table (hand off table) – finger flexors and thumb abductors forearm supinated. Finger extensors and thumb adductors forearm pronated
Finger abductors and adductors and thumb extensors and flexors (movement in sagittal plane)	Supine or sitting	Supine or sitting with forearm in pronation	Supine or sitting at hand table (hand off table) – thumb flexors and finger adductors with shoulder medially rotated and forearm pronated. Thumb extensors and finger abductors forearm in mid position

Therapist For each test, the following protocol should be completed:

1. Position the patient appropriately according to the grade and muscle action.
2. Demonstrate the movement being assessed to the patient.
3. Explain the procedure.
4. Carry out the test for each specific grade (instruction given below).
5. Record the grade.
6. Compare with the other side of the body.

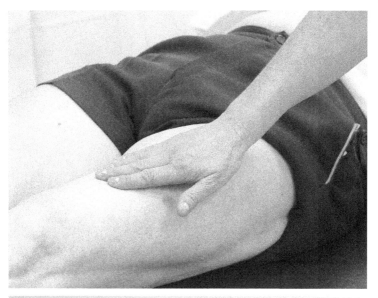

Figure 30.2 Oxford muscle grading for knee extension: Grades 0 and 1.

Testing for grade 0 and 1

1. Ask the patient to attempt to either contract the muscle in a static position or attempt to move the limb in an appropriate direction related to the muscles function. The use of words such as 'tighten or squeeze' should inform the patient of what is required.
2. Observe and palpate the muscle in question (Fig. 30.2).
   Can the patient produce any contraction of the target muscle? If no, grade as 0. If there is a flicker of contraction grade 1 is recorded. If the patient produces a movement or strong contraction, move on to test for grade 2.

Testing for grade 2

1. The therapist needs to consider a suitable position so that the movement is:
   a. Through the full ROM. For example, full extension of the hip starts at full hip flexion and ends at full hip extension
   b. Not being *assisted or resisted* by gravity
   c. Isolated. This may require the therapist to support the weight of the limb being tested, e.g. when assessing the hip abductors.

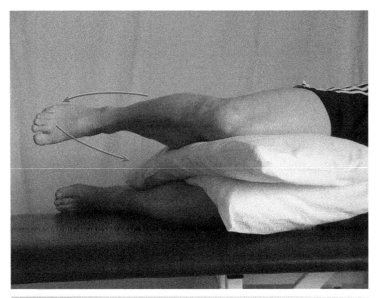

Figure 30.3 Oxford muscle grading for knee extension: Grade 2.

2. Ask the patient to 'Move the body part from start position to finish position' (Fig. 30.3).
   Can the patient move through the full ROM? If no, grade as 1. If yes, they are graded 2 and the therapist should move on to test for grade 3.

 Caution
Manual handling risk: Supporting the weight of a limb.
Risk management: (1) Raise the bed height to a height which is comfortable and which allows you to maintain an upright posture. (2) Keep knees soft to move around your base easily. (3) Maintain a secure hold of the limb.

Testing for grade 3
   1. The therapist needs to consider a suitable position so that the movement is:
      a. Through the full ROM
      b. Being *resisted* by gravity. With some muscle actions, it is not possible to carry out the full ROM against gravity in one

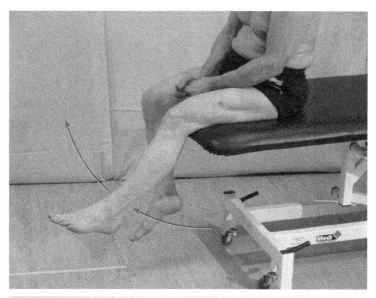

Figure 30.4 Oxford muscle grading for knee extension: Grade 3.

movement. In these cases, a second posture should be sought in order to test the action in two halves. For example, to test shoulder flexion – supine with upper limb off the edge of the plinth to test full extension to neutral and in standing to test neutral to full flexion.

2. Ask the patient to 'Move the body part from start position to finish position' (Fig. 30.4).

Can the patient achieve full ROM against gravity? If no, grade 2 is allocated. If yes, they are graded 3 and the therapist should move on to test for grade 4.

Testing for grade 4

1. The therapist needs to consider a suitable position so that the movement is:
   a. Through the full ROM
   b. Being *resisted* by gravity
   c. Additional 'minimal resistance' is provided throughout the ROM by the therapist. The therapist needs to consider how much resistance to use relating to 'minimal' and should modify the resistance applied according to the size of muscle

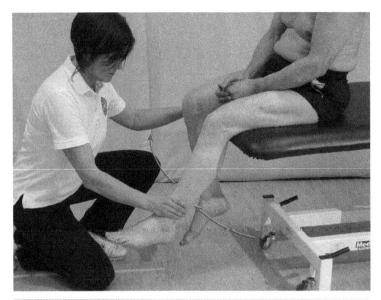

Figure 30.5 Oxford muscle grading for knee extension: Grades 4 and 5.

being tested and the patient's characteristics (e.g. age and gender).

2. Note: In clinical practice, the application of an additional resistance through the ROM is often considered to negate the need for the action to be against gravity.

3. Ask the patient to 'Move the body part from start position to finish position'.

4. Apply minimal resistance throughout the full ROM (Fig. 30.5). *Can the patient achieve full ROM against a minimal resistance applied by the therapist?* If no, grade 3 is awarded. If yes, grade 4 is recorded and the therapist should move on to test grade 5.

 Caution

Manual handling risk: Working away from your body.

   Risk management: In order to support the weight of a limb or resist certain muscle actions through the full ROM the therapist should assess one half of the range standing one side of the plinth and then move to the other side of the plinth to assess the other half of the range.

Testing for grade 5

1. The therapist needs to consider a suitable position so that the movement is:
   a. Through the full ROM
   b. Being *resisted* by gravity. Note the point made in grade 4 section
   c. Additional 'maximal resistance' is provided throughout the ROM by the therapist. Grade 5 represents normal strength, however maximal resistance will need to be adapted according to which muscle action is being tested and other patient specific factors.
2. Ask the patient to 'Move the body part from the start position to the finish position'.
3. Apply maximal resistance throughout the full ROM (Fig. 30.5).
   Can the patient achieve full ROM against maximal resistance? If no, grade 4 is given. If yes, record grade 5.

Caution
Manual handling risk: The application of resistance to the muscle action (grades 4 and 5). Some muscle groups (knee extensors) will impose a greater risk than others (wrist extensors).
Risk management: The therapist should be positioned to gain the greatest mechanical advantage during the test so reducing the effort required and to improve patient comfort. This may be achieved by applying the resistance at the end of a lever (limb), using your body weight as resistance and ensuring that you have a stable base that is elongated in the direction that you will need to move.

Clinical hints and tips
If during tests for grade 2–5 the patient is only able to complete full ROM using trick movements, this may represent weakness or a poor motor control strategy. Further investigation is required or a repeat of the test with stricter instructions and allocation of a lower grade.

RECORDING

The grade awarded is usually recorded in relation to the total possible score. For example grade 4 strength is notated as 4/5. A simple table (Table 30.3) or a list of results allowing comparison

Table 30.3 Example of recording manual muscle testing

	Left	Right
Shoulder extensors	4/5	5/5
Shoulder flexors	4/5	5/5
Shoulder abductors	3/5	5/5
Shoulder adductors	3/5	5/5

of left and right sides of the body is acceptable and gives a clear and easily understandable record of the findings.

ANALYSIS

A comparison of scores for left and right sides of the body is the first step of analysis. However, if the impairment of strength is suspected to be bilateral, as in the case of Guillain–Barré syndrome and motor neuron disease, this analysis will be invalid. In this situation, a comparison can only be made against the therapist's expectation of what 'normal strength' would be for that individual person. Any score below 5/5 is indicative of muscle weakness and should be targeted as requiring a strengthening programme.

In the above example, the left shoulder muscles are generally weaker than the right in the directions identified.

OUTCOME MEASURE

RESEARCH
The gold standard for assessing muscle strength is isokinetic dynamometry, which measures isokinetic muscle strength (e.g. Cybex (Medway, MA) and KinCom (IsoKinetic International, Harrison, TN). However, the clinical usefulness of such machines is limited by their cost and size. The hand held dynamometer is more realistic for use in a clinical setting but only provides an objective measure for isometric muscle strength.

CLINICAL
- Oxford grading (MRC scale)
- Motricity Index
- Hand held dynamometer.

REFERENCES AND FURTHER READING

Ada L, Dorsch S, Canning CG: Strengthening interventions increase strength and improve activity after CVA: a systematic review, *Australian Journal of Physiotherapy* 52:241–248, 2006.

Brown DA, Kautz SA: Increased workload enhances force output during pedaling exercise in persons with post-CVA hemiplegia, *Stroke* 29:598–606, 1998.

Badics E, Wittmann A, Rupp M: Systematic muscle building exercises in the rehabilitation of CVA patients, *NeuroRehabilitation* 17:211–214, 2002.

Bale M, Strand LI: Does functional strength training of the leg in subacute stroke improve physical performance? A pilot randomized controlled trial, *Clinical Rehabilitation* 22(10–11):911–921, 2008.

Chae J, Yang G, Park BK, et al: Muscle weakness and cocontraction in upper limb hemiparesis: relationship to motor impairment and physical disability, *Neurorehabilitation and Neural Repair* 16:241–248, 2002.

Dyck PJ, Boes CJ, Mulder D, et al: History of standard scoring notation and summation of neuromuscular signs: a current survey and recommendation, *Journal of the Peripheral Nervous System* 10:158–173, 2005.

Hara Y, Akaboshi K, Masakado Y, et al: Physiologic decrease of single thenar motor units in the F-response in CVA patients, *Archives of Physical Medicine and Rehabilitation* 81:418–423, 2000.

Kim CM, Eng JJ: The relationship of lower-extremity muscle torque to locomotor performance in people with CVA, *Physical Therapy* 83:49–57, 2003.

Knuttgen H, Kraemer W: Terminology and measurement in exercise performance, *Journal of Applied Sport Science and Research* 1:1–10, 1987.

Kraemer WJ, Adams K, Cafarelli E, et al: American College of Sports Medicine position stand. Progression models in resistance training for healthy adults, *Medicine and Science in Sports and Exercise* 34:364–380, 2002.

Lieber RL: *Skeletal muscle structure, function and plasticity: the physiological basis of rehabilitation,* ed 2, Philadelphia, 2002, Lippincott Williams and Wilkins.

Medical Research Council (MRC): *Aids to the investigation of the peripheral nervous system*, London, 1976, Her Majesty's Stationery Office.

Mercier C, Bourbonnais D: Relative shoulder flexor and handgrip strength is related to upper limb function after CVA, *Clinical Rehabilitation* 18:215–221, 2004.

Moore DP, Kowalske KJ: Neuromuscular rehabilitation and electrodiagnosis of myopathy, *Archives of Physical Medicine and Rehabilitation* 81:S32–S35, 2000.

Morris SL, Dodd KJ, Morris ME: Outcomes of progressive resistance strength training following CVA: a systematic review, *Clinical Rehabilitation* 18:27–39, 2004.

Palastanga N, Field D, Soames R: *Anatomy and human movement: structure and function,* ed 5, Edinburgh, 2006, Butterworth Heinemann/ Elsevier.

Ryan AS, Dobrovolny CL, Smith GV, et al: Hemiparetic muscle atrophy and increased intramuscular fat in CVA patients, *Archives of Physical Medicine and Rehabilitation* 83:1703–1707, 2002.

Sharp SA, Brouwer BJ: Isokinetic strength training of the hemiparetic knee: effects on function and spasticity, *Archives of Physical Medicine and Rehabilitation* 78:1231–1236, 1997.

Sterr A, Freivogel S: Intensive training in chronic upper limb hemiparesis does not increase spasticity or synergies, *Neurology* 63:2176–2177, 2004.

Taylor NF, Dodd KJ, Prasad D, et al: Progressive resistance exercise for people with multiple sclerosis, *Disability and Rehabilitation* 2818:1119–1126, 2006.

Weiss A, Suzuki T, Bean J, et al: High intensity strength training improves strength and functional performance after CVA, *American Journal of Physical Medicine and Rehabilitation* 794:369–376, 2000.

Yang Y-R, Wang R-Y, Lin K-H, et al: Task-oriented progressive resistance strength training improves muscle strength and functional performance in individuals with stroke, *Clinical Rehabilitation* 20:860–870, 2006.

Myotomes

WHAT IS A MYOTOME?

A myotome is defined as the group of muscles supplied by one spinal nerve root level. There are 31 pairs of spinal nerves (S2.13) each contributing to the innervations of many muscles (e.g. C_5 innervates parts of supraspinatus, infraspinatus, deltoid and biceps). The muscles supplied by a single nerve root level are generally involved in a common muscle action/s and it is this muscle action that is assessed. The list below identifies a simplified version of the actions associated with each spinal nerve root level (Grieve 2004).

C1/C2 – neck flexion/neck extension (see Fig. 31.1)
C3 – neck side flexion
C4 – shoulder elevation
C5 – shoulder abduction (see Fig. 31.2)
C6 – elbow flexion or forearm supination
C7 – elbow extension or wrist flexion
C8 – thumb extension or adduction and ulna deviation
T1 – finger abduction/adduction
L2 – hip flexion or adduction
L3 – knee extension (see Fig. 31.3)
L4 – dorsi flexion at the ankle
L5 – big toe extension or ankle eversion
S1 – plantar flexion of the ankle or knee flexion.

WHY DO I NEED TO ASSESS MYOTOMES?

Assessing a myotome gives information related to nerve integrity, in other words, whether the nerve pathway from the spinal cord to the muscle is intact. The assessment evaluates the strength of the muscle contraction, however it should be remembered that a weak muscle could be the result of a lesion anywhere along the nerve pathway but also of the muscle itself. Knowledge of the muscles supplied by the spinal nerve root (myotome) and the peripheral nerve allows the therapist to differentiate between lesions of each (Petty 2006). A complete lesion of the peripheral nerve will lead to complete paralysis of the muscles innervated by that nerve. Therefore, weakness will be evident immediately on testing and muscle atrophy will occur over time. However, the presentation of a lesion to a single nerve root will be more difficult to recognize because the muscle itself will still be innervated by other unaffected root levels within the peripheral nerve. For example, the biceps muscle is supplied by the musculocutaneous nerve ($C_{5/6/7}$). Therefore, any lesion affecting C_6 nerve root will present as minor weakness because sufficient motor units can be recruited via the remaining root levels $C_{5/7}$. However, if the therapist provides resistance over a period of time (5–10 seconds) the weakness may become evident.

Caution

A motor loss related to a single myotome may be indicative of a lesion at the spinal nerve root but must be confirmed by a similar finding for that particular root level for dermatomes (S3.24) and reflexes (S3.22).

In terms of neurologically impaired patients, the clinical presentation of any motor loss *only* requires assessment using myotomes when there is involvement of either the spinal cord specifically or the peripheral nervous system, e.g. spinal cord injury (SCI) and Guillain–Barré syndrome (GBS). As neither of these pathologies affects the spinal nerve root in isolation, myotome testing is less clinically useful as a diagnostic tool, however it is a very useful way of mapping the motor loss. The map produced gives the therapist a highly relevant outcome measure, by which the extent and level of motor loss can first be estimated and then re-evaluated. This is especially important in recovering conditions, such as GBS and in SCI, where a rising level of motor loss may reflect a serious deterioration of the injury.

HOW DO I ASSESS A MYOTOME?

Patient

For testing the upper limb, the posture of sitting should be acceptable. To complete the lower limb assessment sitting, supine or prone may be necessary.

Therapist

1. Identify a muscle action from the list above.
2. Resistance is applied by the therapist so that the muscles being assessed contract isometrically. Therefore no movement should occur at the joint which may confound the findings.
3. Where possible the test should be performed in middle range of the action (Figs 31.1–31.3).
4. The resistance should be brought on slowly to allow the patient to build up to the level of resistance offered by the therapist.
5. The amount of force applied should be appropriate to the size of the muscle being tested, especially for neck movements.

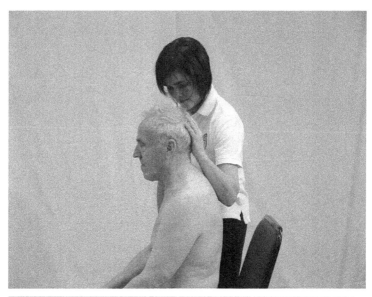

Figure 31.1 Testing for myotome C3.

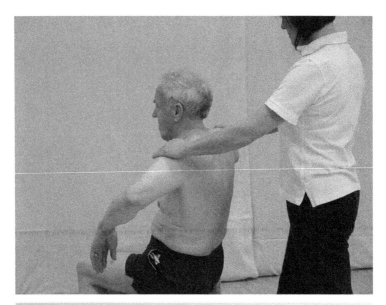

Figure 31.2 Testing for myotome C5.

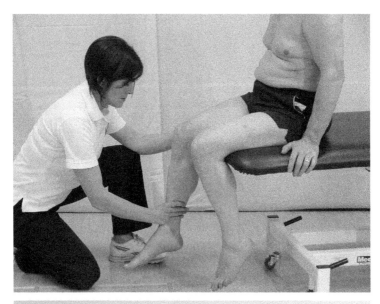

Figure 31.3 Testing for myotome L3.

6. The isometric contraction should be held for approximately 5–10 seconds.
7. Where possible, the left and right sides should be compared simultaneously (Fig. 31.2).

  Is there weakness evident in the action? Yes, there may be a deficit within the peripheral nervous system. If other spinal root levels appear intact the deficit may be localized to the root level being tested and should be confirmed using evidence from dermatome and reflex testing for the same level. However, if the distribution of loss is more generalized, this is unlikely to be the case.

  Is the strength of contraction the same on both sides? No, this could indicate a unilateral deficit.

RECORDING

The therapist should note all the muscle actions that present with weakness. A simple statement of what was assessed and a list of abnormal findings is sufficient. In the case of GBS and SCI, the loss may be extensive but detailed analysis is crucial and may be easier to record on a body chart.

Example
All myotomes assessed:

Upper limbs: Nothing abnormal detected (NAD) and left side = right side
Lower limbs: Left L3 presents with weakness. Nil else of note.

ANALYSIS

The findings of weakness related to a single myotome should be analysed along with any abnormal findings from dermatome testing and reflexes. The findings from all three assessments can be used to identify specifically the level and extent of a lesion or if relevant to differentiate a spinal nerve root deficit.

OUTCOME MEASURE

Research and clinically
Myotome testing is viewed as an outcome measure to be used as an ongoing tool for evaluation.

REFERENCES

Grieve GP: *Grieve's modern manual therapy: the vertebral column*, ed 3, Edinburgh, 2004, Churchill Livingstone.

Petty NJ: *Neuromusculoskeletal examination and assessment: a handbook for therapists*, ed 3, Edinburgh, 2006, Churchill Livingstone/Elsevier.

Balance

WHAT IS BALANCE?

In biomechanical terms, balance is a state whereby the projection of the centre of mass (COM) falls within the stability limits of the base of support (BOS). The stability limit being the point at which balance is lost and corrective action is required. Balance is a core component of all functional activities and as such, incorporates both the concepts of posture (arrested movement) and movement. The control of posture and movement in attaining a state of balance is often termed *postural control* and describes the motor action that occurs following the integration of sensory, perceptual, cognitive and motor processes. The aims of postural control are:

- *Postural equilibrium/stability* involving the coordination of movement strategies to:
  - Maintain an upright posture against gravity and any other external forces

- Maintain the COM within the stability limits of the BOS during internally and externally initiated movement (planned/intentional and unpredictable).
- *Postural orientation* involving the control of body segment alignment with respect to:
  - Gravity
  - Vertical
  - Internal references
  - The environment (Horak 2006).

SENSORY INPUT AND BALANCE

The state of balance is maintained through complex postural control mechanisms which are reliant on adequate sensory input. The principal input systems to balance are the vestibular system (S2.10), the visual system (S2.10) and the somatosensory systems (S3.23) (Massion et al. 2004). Visual input provides a reference for upright vertical but is also essential in predicting forthcoming threats to balance from the environment. The somatosensory system, primarily proprioception, provides a reference for the body's position in relation to the supporting surface and to other body parts and finally the vestibular system provides a reference for head position and movement of the head in relation to gravity.

In general this sensory input has two main functions:

Sensory feed forward which allows a preparation for movement. These anticipatory adjustments require input from both the internal and external environment and are an integral part of every movement. They are strongly linked to previous experiences.

Sensory feedback which allows ongoing regulation and appropriate muscle adjustments to be made in response to planned and unplanned displacement of the COM during movement.

INTEGRATION

Integration of this sensory information for an appropriate motor response is facilitated by various higher centres, including: the brain stem and cranial nerves (S2.10); the cerebellum (S2.12); reticular formation (S2.10) and the cerebral cortex (S2.7). The amount of cognitive processing by the cortex for postural control is usually minimal, with its contribution depending on the complexity of the task and the capability of the individual's postural control system. For example, postural control relies on accurate sensory input, but also on the ability of the central nervous system

(CNS) to attend to the relevant sensory cues and to prioritize or weight the input according to its relevance to the context and task (Horak 2006). The CNS also intervenes if a sensory conflict exists when it must weight the sources and reject the potential source of error (Karnath et al. 2000b).

MOTOR OUTPUT AND BALANCE

During movement there is inevitably a displacement of the COM in relation to the BOS. This occurs whether the movement involves the trunk, the upper limb, the lower limb, turning the head or simply breathing. What determines whether the displacement leads to a fall is the motor response by which balance is recovered. These motor adjustments are flexible and varied and dependent on the task, the environmental context and the individual. An appropriate motor response requires a certain level of muscle strength, endurance and an available range of movement (Cholewicki et al. 1997; Ebenbichler and Oddsson 2001; Hodges and Richardson 1997) but also fine grading of agonists, antagonists and synergistic muscles, appropriate co-contraction and a high level of reciprocal innervation.

Although postural control mechanisms are varied, certain patterns of activation are described, however in an adult these are integrated into movement and may not always be evident:

Movement strategies

An individual can slow down the displacement of the COM by rapidly generating muscle torque at the ankles, hips or other joints around a fixed BOS. For anteroposterior displacements of the COM the predominant torque is generated via an ankle strategy (Fig. 32.1) although a hip strategy (Fig. 32.2) may also be present. For a mediolateral displacement, the hip strategy is dominant (Maki and McIlroy 2006). These strategies occur in a feed forward manner to maintain balance and are continuously interchangeable during movement. However, if the perturbation is large and these strategies are unsuccessful, the individual may actually change the BOS by stepping (Fig. 32.3) or using an outstretched arm. Although the latter response is often referred to as protective it can also occur during small perturbations as a normal strategy for balance.

Balance reactions

Equilibrium reactions These are subtle changes in muscle tone required to *maintain* equilibrium and are analogous with postural sway (Fig. 32.4). When people stand with their eyes closed, postural sway may increase by 20–70% (Lord and Menz 2000).

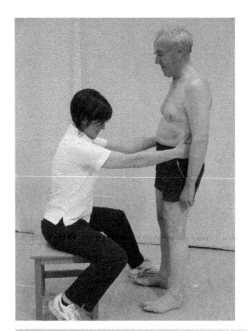

Figure 32.1 Movement strategy: Ankle.

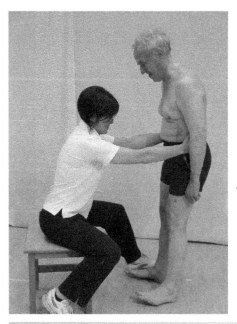

Figure 32.2 Movement strategy: Hip.

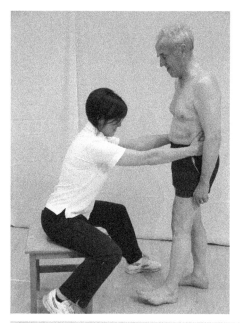

Figure 32.3 Movement strategy: Step backwards.

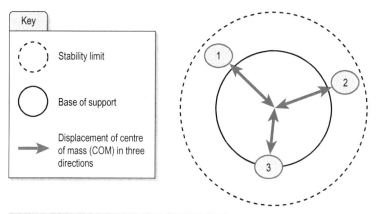

Key

- - - Stability limit

◯ Base of support

⟶ Displacement of centre of mass (COM) in three directions

Figure 32.4 Equilibrium reactions.

Righting reactions The existence of righting reactions in a mature adult is debated as it is proposed that they become integrated with equilibrium reactions by age 3 months. However, as the debate appears to be one of terminology and is as yet unresolved, this text describes the two phenomena separately.

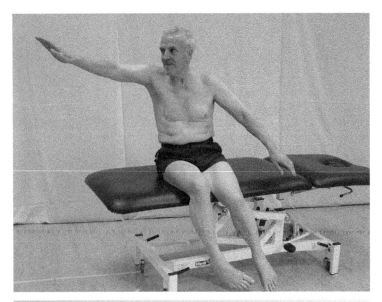

Figure 32.5 Righting reactions in sitting.

Righting reactions occur in response to displacement of the COM beyond the stability limits in an attempt to *regain* equilibrium. They are a basic component in maintaining equilibrium while changing between positions and hence during movement. Righting reactions may involve the head (moving on the trunk to maintain the head in vertical), the trunk (in response to weight transfer or head/limb movement) or limb movement (acting as a counter balance to offset the displacement of COM) (Fig. 32.5). *Saving/protective* When the displacement of the COM is beyond the stability limits and righting reactions are inadequate a step or an extended upper limb may be used in order that a new base of support is established and equilibrium restored.

WHY DO WE NEED TO ASSESS BALANCE?

Balance impairments have been shown to increase the risk of falls (S3.34) resulting in high economic costs and social problems (Lamb et al. 2003; Harris et al. 2005; Belgen et al. 2006). Balance problems in neurologically impaired patients are common, being associated with the following impairments:

MOTOR DYSFUNCTION

Musculoskeletal

- Decreased muscle strength: In cerebrovascular accident (CVA) (Belgen et al. 2006; Tyson et al. 2006; Au-Yeung et al. 2003; Niam et al. 1999)
- Trunk instability: In CVA (Verheyden et al. 2006; Karatas et al. 2004)
- Decreased range of movement
- Altered muscle tone.

Biomechanics

- Reduced stability limits: In CVA (De Haart et al. 2004) and in Parkinson's disease (PD) (Mancini et al. 2008)
- Reduced balance response (magnitude and velocity): In PD (Mancini et al. 2008)
- Altered movement strategies: In CVA there is a reliance on hip and stepping strategies which are less efficient in terms of stability (Maki and McIlroy 1997; Chen et al. 2000).

SENSORY DYSFUNCTION

Altered sensation

- Deceased ankle proprioception: In CVA (Tyson et al. 2006) and in PD (Vaugoyeau et al. 2007)
- Vestibular system damage
- Dizziness
- Visual deficits.

Altered sensory integration

- Difficulty dividing attention between two tasks (Stapleton et al. 2001)
- Impaired ability to use sensory weighting: Reduced speed of integration in PD (Brown et al. 2006; De Nunzio et al. 2007). In CVA there is often excessive reliance on visual input which may lead to inappropriate postural adjustments (Bonan et al. 2004)
- Delayed or inadequate anticipatory response: In CVA and PD (Horak et al. 1997)
- Altered perceived stability limits: In CVA (De Haart et al. 2004) linked to anxiety and lack of confidence
- Abnormal perception of vertical via the somatosensory systems in CVA, particularly in association with visuospatial neglect (Yelnik et al. 2002; Bonan et al. 2006).

Clinical hints and tips

It is interesting that in healthy subjects our perceived stability limit and the consequent motor response may be altered if we fear a threat to our balance (e.g. icy ground or wet floor). This is highly relevant in patients who readily lose confidence and as a consequence, they may limit themselves functionally over time.

HOW DO I ASSESS BALANCE?

The state of balance is primarily a background to performing a movement and in the main is automatically controlled. Therefore it should be assessed in this context, that is, during performance of a task or function. However, several options are available to the therapist.

FUNCTIONAL OBSERVATION

Patient

In order to assess balance in context the patient should be requested to perform a functional activity. The choice of activity will be dependent on the patient's ability.

Therapist

1. The therapist should set an appropriate balance task. When setting a task the therapist should consider the following:
   a. Create a safe situation (environment, assistance as required).
   b. Incorporate various environmental contexts and various tasks as our postural control is highly specific to both.
   c. Challenge their balance: This means making them unstable and could be achieved by:
      - Reducing the size of the base of support
      - Raising the COM
      - Displacing the COM towards the stability limits by either a movement created by the therapist or the patient. If the patient is unstable requesting them to turn their head may be challenge enough
      - Placing them on an unstable surface
      - Alter their sensory input: Use eyes open and eyes closed.
   d. Assess all aspects of balance responses:
      - Posture and movement
      - Balance strategies: ankle, hip and step

- Balance reactions: equilibrium/righting and saving
- Different planes of movement (transverse, sagittal and frontal planes).

2. Observe the patient performing the balance task.

Can they balance (maintain the COM within the BOS) in a specific posture? Instability during a stable posture may indicate a severe balance deficit. If there is inappropriate excessive sway in all postures with eyes open, then sufficient assistance is recommended before challenging the patient any further.

Can they balance during movement? If not, do they fall?

If they can balance, what strategies do they use to achieve balance? Are their responses appropriate for the amount of COM displacement?

Does the patient use compensatory strategies to maintain balance? Using trunk or limb muscles to fix is inefficient and may indicate underlying instability. Visual fixation is also common.

Are these compensations effective?

Is the goal completed successfully? Without a stable/balanced base the execution may be unsuccessful.

Is the task performance effortful? This may indicate extra muscle work to hide poor balance.

Do they interact with their BOS during the movement? The BOS should act as a point of reference for movement. The base providing a stable point that the patient can move around confidently.

What happens to the balance if sensory input is reduced (e.g. eyes closed)?

SPECIAL TESTS: ROMBERG'S TEST

Therapist

1. The patient is asked to begin in tandem stance (feet heel to toe) with eyes open.
2. This is held for 5–10 seconds.
3. The test is repeated with eyes closed.
4. The therapist should observe the amount of postural sway in both conditions.

Is there an increased postural sway exhibited when the eyes are open and closed? This is indicative of a deficit of the cerebellum.

Is there normal postural sway with eyes open which excessively deteriorates when eyes are closed? This is attributed to a somatosensory deficit.

RECORDING

A simple text description of the therapist's assessment and findings is sufficient. This should include the patient's functional ability to balance and some description related to the quality of the motor response.

Example
Balance:
    Patient is sitting – Pt is able to sit unsupported for a limited time (10 seconds) and maintains this posture using excessive activity around both hips. Postural sway is normal.
    Patient was able to lift both hands off his lap for approx. 2 seconds, during which he became anxious. Further assessment was inappropriate.

ANALYSIS

Postural control is hugely complex and therefore simple balance measures are unlikely to identify the specific deficits of the senso-rimotor processes. Comprehensive assessment is required to eval-uate the potential impairments implicated in a deficit of balance. Therefore the findings from your balance assessment must be considered in conjunction with the findings from other assess-ment tools (S3.19–34). Particular attention should be paid to vision (S3.27) and sensory testing (S3.23) and if a lesion of the vestibular system is suspected, referral to a specialist unit is advised. However, trunk stability, muscle tone, alignment, pain, strength, range of movement and cognition/perception may also be linked to reduced balance.
    In the above example, the patient maintains balance in sitting using an ineffective compensatory strategy. His underlying balance deficit is related to hypotonia of his trunk, based on other find-ings. He also appears to have developed an altered perception of his stability limits as he becomes anxious without apparent need. This could limit the voluntary use of his upper limbs in the future.

OUTCOME MEASURES

RESEARCH
Posturography refers to any technique used to quantify postural control in standing. These objective quantitative measures of

balance can assess with greater sensitivity than observation by the therapist (De Oliveira 2008). Postural reactions can be quantified on force platforms with the sensory environment being manipulated to challenge different systems of balance. However, the output from a force platform does not tell the therapist about the quality of the postural control mechanisms.

CLINICAL

- Tinetti balance
- Berg balance scale
- Romberg's test
- Sharpened Romberg's
- Functional reach test
- Functional activities: validated in stroke (Tyson and DeSouza 2004)
- Sitting: supported sitting balance, sitting arm raise, sitting forward reach
- Standing: supported standing balance, standing arm raise, standing forward reach, static tandem standing, weight shift
- Walking: timed 5-m walk with and without an aid, tap and step.

REFERENCES AND FURTHER READING

Au-Yeung SS, Ng JT, Lo SK: Does balance or motor impairment of limbs discriminate the ambulatory status of stroke survivors? *American Journal of Physical Medicine and Rehabilitation* 824:279–283, 2003.

Belgen B, Beninato M, Sullivan PE, et al: The association of balance capacity and falls self-efficacy with history of falling in community-dwelling people with chronic stroke, *Archives of Physical Medicine and Rehabilitation* 874:554–561, 2006.

Bonan IV, Colle FM, Guichard JP, et al: Reliance on visual information after stroke, Part I: Balance on dynamic posturography, *Archives of Physical Medicine Rehabilitation* 852:268–273, 2004.

Bonan IV, Guettard E, Leman MC: Subjective visual vertical perception relates to balance in acute stroke, *Archives of Physical Medicine Rehabilitation* 875:642–646, 2006.

Brown LA, Sleik RJ, Winder TR: Attentional demands for static postural control after stroke, *Archives of Physical Medicine Rehabilitation* 8312:1732–1735, 2002.

Brown LA, Cooper SA, Doan JB, et al: Parkinsonian deficits in sensory integration for postural control: temporal response to changes in visual input, *Parkinsonism Related Disorders* 12:376–381, 2006.

Chen IC, Cheng PT, Hu AL, et al: Balance evaluation in hemiplegic stroke patients, *Chan Gung Medical* J236:339–347, 2000.

Cholewicki J, Panjabi M, Khachatryan A: Stabilizing function of trunk flexor and extensor muscles around a neutral spine posture, *Spine* 22:2207–2212, 1997.

Danells CJ, Black SE, Gladstone DJ, et al: Poststroke 'pushing': Natural history and relationship to motor and functional recovery, *Stroke* 3512:2873–2878, 2004.

De Haart M, Geurts AC, Huidekoper SC, et al: Recovery of standing balance in postacute stroke patients: a rehabilitation cohort study, *Archives of Physical Medicine Rehabilitation* 856:886–895, 2004.

De Nunzio AM, Nardone A, Schieppati M: The control of equilibrium in Parkinson's disease patients: delayed adaptation of balancing strategy to shifts in sensory set during a dynamic task, *Brain Research Bulletin* 74:258–270, 2007.

De Oliveira CB, de Medeiros IR, Frota NA, et al: Balance control in hemiparetic stroke patients: main tools for evaluation, *Journal of Rehabilitation Research and Development* 468:1216–1228, 2008.

Ebenbichler G, Oddsson L: Sensory-motor control of the lower back: implications for rehabilitation, *Medicine and Science in Sports and Exercise* 33:1889–1898, 2001.

Garland SJ, Ivanova TD, Mochizuki G: Recovery of standing balance and health-related quality of life after mild or moderately severe stroke, *Archives of Physical Medicine Rehabilitation* 882:218–227, 2007.

Gustafson Y: Falls and injuries after stroke: time for action! *Stroke* 342:494–501, 2003.

Harris JE, Eng JJ, Marigold DS, et al: Relationship of balance and mobility to fall incidence in people with chronic stroke, *Physical Therapy* 852:150–158, 2005.

Hodges P, Richardson C: Relationship between limb movement speed and associated contraction of the trunk muscles, *Ergonomics* 40:1220–1230, 1997.

Horak FB: Postural orientation and equilibrium: what do we need to know about neural control of balance to prevent falls? *Age Ageing* 35(Suppl 2):7–11, 2006.

Horak FB, Henry SM, Shumway-Cook A: Postural perturbations: new insights for treatment of balance disorders, *Physical Therapy* 775:517–533, 1997.

Karnath HO, Broetz D: Understanding and treating 'pusher syndrome', *Physical Therapy* 8312:1119–1125, 2003.

Karnath HO, Ferber S, Dichgans J: The origin of contraversive pushing: evidence for a second graviceptive system in humans, *Neurology* 559:1298–1304, 2000a.

Karnath HO, Ferber S, Dichgans J: The neural representation of postural control in humans, *Proceedings of the National Academy of Science USA* 9725:13931–13936, 2000b.

Karatas M, Cetin N, Bayramoglu M, et al: Trunk muscle strength in relation to balance and functional disability in unihemispheric stroke patients, *American Journal of Physical Medicine and Rehabilitation* 832:81–87, 2004.

Lamb SE, Ferrucci L, Volapto S, et al: Risk factors for falling in home-dwelling older women with stroke: the Women's Health and Aging Study, *Stroke* 342:494–501, 2003.

Lord SR, Menz HB: Visual contributions to postural stability in older adults, *Gerontology* 46:306–310, 2000.

Maki BE, McIlroy WE: The role of limb movements in maintaining upright stance: the 'change-in-support' strategy, *Physical Therapy* 775:488–507, 1997.

Maki BE, McIlroy WE: Control of rapid limb movements for balance recovery: age-related changes and implications for fall prevention, *Age and Ageing* 35-S2:12–18, 2006.

Mancini M, Rocchi L, Horak FB, et al: Effects of Parkinson's disease and levodopa on functional limits of stability, *Clinical Biomechanics* 23:450–458, 2008.

Massion J, Alexandrov A, Frolov A: Why and how are posture and movement coordinated? *Progress in Brain Research* 1432:13–27, 2004.

Niam S, Cheung W, Sullivan PE et al: Balance and physical impairments after stroke, *Archives of Physical Medicine Rehabilitation* 80(10):1227–1233, 1999.

Oie KS, Kiemel T, Jeka JJ: Multisensory fusion: simultaneous re-weighting of vision and touch for the control of human posture, *Brain Research Cognitive Brain Research* 141:164–176, 2002.

Oxford Dictionary. Online. www.askoxford.com/?view=uk.

Peterka JR: Sensorimotor integration in human postural control, *Journal of Neurophysiology* 883:1097–1118, 2002.

Peterka RJ, Loughlin PJ: Dynamic regulation of sensorimotor integration in human postural control, *Journal of Neurophysiology* 911:410–423, 2004.

Stapleton T, Ashburn A, Stack E: A pilot study of attention deficits balance control and falls in the acute stage following stroke, *Clinical Rehabilitation* 15:437–444, 2001.

Stokes M: *Physical management in neurological rehabilitation*, ed 2, Edinburgh, 2004, Elsevier/Mosby.

Tyson SF, DeSouza LH: Reliability and validity of functional balance tests post stroke, *Clinical Rehabilitation* 188:916–923, 2004.

Tyson SF, Hanley M, Chillala J et al: Balance disability after stroke, *Physical Therapy* 861:30–38, 2006.

Vaugoyeau M, Viel S, Assaiante C et al: Impaired vertical postural control and proprioceptive integration deficits in Parkinson's disease, *Neuroscience* 146:852–863, 2007.

Verheyden G, Vereeck L, Truijen S et al: Trunk performance after stroke and the relationship with balance gait and functional ability, *Clinical Rehabilitation* 205:451–458, 2006.

Yelnik AP, Lebreton FO, Bonan IV et al: Perception of verticality after recent cerebral hemispheric stroke, *Stroke* 339:2247–2253, 2002.

Cognition and Perception

WHAT ARE COGNITION AND PERCEPTION?

PERCEPTION

Perception *is* the organization, integration and interpretation of sensory stimuli (S3.23) to provide meaningful information. Perception may not be a direct record of the environment surrounding us because meaning is constructed by our brains based on learning and previous experience and is therefore highly individual. This complex processing involves many areas of the brain including the sensory association areas of the parietal lobe (S2.7).

COGNITION

Cognition is the ability to process, retrieve and manipulate information. Cognition for the most part is localized in the frontal lobe of the cerebral cortex (S2.7), however these specific areas interact with many other areas of the brain, making processing highly complex. Emotion is now also considered a cognitive process.

Perception and cognitive functions are essential for efficient interaction with our environment and have been found to have an impact on both movement and posture with impairments noted as a poor prognostic indicator in the population of neurologically impaired patients. The list below shows the hierarchical arrangement of normal perceptual and cognitive processes. Note that the higher levels of the hierarchy depend upon the lower levels as part of their construct:

● Executive function
● Praxis
● Recognition
● Memory
● Body schema
● Basic perception
● Attention
● Sensory registration.

Sensory registration

This incorporates the ability to receive and modulate sensory information and is a prerequisite for perception. Patients with a sensory impairment are therefore likely to experience some perceptual/cognitive problems.

Attention

This ability is related to how we become receptive to our sensory environment and allows us to restrict our attention to what is relevant at the present time. This is vital when considering the constant bombardment of our sensory systems. Deficits related to attention are usually associated with damage to the right hemisphere and common presentations include poor attention span and being easily distracted.

Five levels of attention have been identified:

Focused attention: The ability to focus on one stimulus

Sustained attention: The ability to maintain attention over a period of time, often referred to as attention span

Selective attention: The ability to focus on a specific stimulus, while filtering out any non-relevant stimuli (distractions)

Switching attention: The ability to switch focus between two or more stimuli

Divided attention: The ability to respond to more than one stimulus at one time. For example, talking while walking. This ability is easier when the stimuli are from different sensory modalities.

Basic perception

This includes the processing/interpretation of all sensory modalities:

Touch perception (stereognosis): This is the ability to interpret information using only tactile and proprioceptive sensation.

Visual perception:

Visual processing allows us to interpret and organize visual information. This processing occurs primarily in the visual association areas of the occipital, parietal and temporal lobes (S2.7) (Kandel et al. 2000). There are two main aspects to visual perception:

Visuoperceptual: This involves the interpretation of the form of an object, such as colour, texture, shape, size and includes size and form constancy. Form and size constancy are the ability to recognize the same object even when it is in a different context or of a different size.

Visuospatial: This involves the interpretation of spatial relationships such as depth, distance, up/down, in/out, left/right, 2D/3D, figure ground. Figure ground is the ability to differentiate foreground from background. For example, this ability is necessary to distinguish the keys when dialling a number on a telephone key pad or using a TV remote control. Impairments of visuospatial perception can include topographic disorientation (difficulty with orientating between places), poor figure ground and visuospatial neglect.

Visuospatial neglect is the inability to report, respond or integrate sensory stimuli on the contralateral side of the body to the brain lesion (Shumway-Cook and Woollacott 2007). It is important to understand that this is not a deficit of the visual system but a perceptual impairment usually as a result of right hemisphere lesion (National Clinical Guidelines for Stroke 2004). In its mildest form, the patient may just be inattentive to one side and with instruction/encouragement can scan to the affected side. However, in severe cases, the patient may be completely unaware of any sensory stimuli on the affected side and cannot be encouraged to scan. In this case, the person may be witnessed to only eat food from one half of a plate and will not acknowledge anyone who approaches from the affected side.

Body schema

Body schema is defined as the internal picture which informs our awareness of body parts and their relative position to each other and the environment. It provides a basis for exploration and motor performance. It is continually distributed to networks that plan movement and is updated on a moment by moment basis. A deficit of body schema may result in asomatognosia (the inability to recognize body parts and their relative relationships), visuospatial neglect, left right discrimination or anosognosia (denial of the existence of a disability) (Shumway-Cook and Woollacott 2007). These impairments may lead to problems with mobility and activities of daily living. A further complication is 'pusher syndrome'.

A *pusher* resists weight bearing on their non-affected side due to a fear of falling in that direction (Karnath et al 2007). Studies indicate the cause of this syndrome is an altered perception of vertical via the somatosensory systems and ultimately body schema. Interestingly, there appears to be no disturbed processing determining visual vertical (Broetz and Karnath 2005).

Memory

A memory is a specific synchronous pattern of neuronal activity, termed an engram, which occurs as a consequence of learning. Memory involves three stages: encoding, storage and recall, and as such any deficit may result in problems taking on new information or remembering and retrieving learned information. Memories are processed and stored in various regions of the brain and this reflects the existence of different types of memory:

- *Sensory memory*: This allows us to hold a large amount of information for 1–2 seconds.
- *Short-term/working memory*: This allows 7 ± 2 bits of information to be held between 30–60 seconds.
- *Long-term memory*: This potentially has an unlimited capacity and consists of various types of memory:
  - *Declarative memory* stored primarily in the medial temporal lobe in the limbic association areas and comprises:
    - *Episodic memory* of time and place (e.g. what I had for breakfast)
    - *Semantic memory* of general knowledge
  - *Autobiographical memory*: related to our life events.
  - *Procedural memory*: this is our motor memory, often termed implicit memory. Stored in the cerebellum and supplementary and pre motor areas of the frontal lobe.
  - *Prospective memory*: for future events. For example, remembering birthdays.

Recognition

This requires the integration of sensory registration, attention, visual perception and memory to recognize an object, face, etc. and attach meaning. Agnosia is the loss of this ability which may involve recognition of objects, persons, sounds, shapes, or smells.

Praxis

This is the ability to produce skilled purposeful movement. It basically consists of the conceptual ability to organize the task (ideation) and the ability to apply the motor programme correctly (ideomotor). Dyspraxia is a disorder of praxis and is of five types: verbal, facial/oral, limb, constructional and dressing. Dyspraxia is associated with both left and right hemisphere damage, but more commonly with a left sided neurological lesion (National Clinical Guidelines for Stroke 2004; Shumway-Cook and Woollacott 2007).

Limb dyspraxia is defined by two extremes: ideational and ideomotor. However, it is important to note that a continuum exists between the two and patients often present with elements of both conditions. Diagnosis is usually based upon a movement disorder that cannot be explained by any other impairment (e.g. altered tone, sensory loss or incoordination).

Ideational dyspraxia may present with the elements of the task performed in the wrong order; being omitted from the sequence; two or more elements blended together; or with the sequence of actions not completed. The task *cannot* be performed automatically or with command.

Ideomotor dyspraxia may present as an altered trajectory of movement; poor distance judgement; gestural enhancement; perseveration; vocal overflow; or with a body part being used as an object. The task *can* be performed automatically but not on command.

Higher executive function

This function includes planning, organization, problem-solving, self-initiation, self-monitoring and self-inhibition of behaviour, and is associated with the frontal lobes of the cerebral cortex (S2.7). The ability to learn is also a cognitive skill and therapists rely heavily on both implicit (during motor learning) and explicit learning (when giving instructions) in rehabilitation. A deficit of these higher level cognitive skills is often termed dys-executive syndrome and may include the behaviours indicated in Table 33.1.

Table 33.1 Behaviours associated with dysexecutive syndrome

Executive skill	Abnormal behaviour
Initiation drive	Apathy and unable to initiate behaviour
Response inhibition	Impulsive and over responsive. Perseveration
Task persistence	Unable to maintain attention
Organize actions and thoughts	Problems identifying goals and planning behaviour
Generative thinking	Rigid and narrow thinking. Limited creativity and flexibility
Awareness of own behaviour	Difficulty modifying behaviour. Limited insight into actions, feelings and deficits

WHY DO I NEED TO CONSIDER COGNITION AND PERCEPTION?

In pathologies that may affect the cerebral cortex and higher centres, cognitive and perceptual deficits are common and potentially as debilitating as any physical symptom.

The incidence in Parkinson's disease (PD) is high, although not viewed as a primary symptom of the disease. Dysexecutive syndrome (Demakis 2007), visuospatial dysfunction and change in memory and mood (The Parkinson's Disease Society 2007) have been reported in early PD, with long-term survivors likely to develop dementia.

The incidence in multiple sclerosis (MS) is reported as 50–80% (MS Resource Centre 2002), with the most common symptoms being mild problems with memory, attention span and the speed of processing information. Factors that exacerbate these deficits include low mood and depression, stress, heat and fatigue.

The incidence in cerebrovascular accident (CVA) is also high and commonly constitutes a lack of spatial awareness, poor attention span and problems with memory and higher executive function (National Clinical Guidelines for Stroke 2004).

HOW DO I SCREEN FOR COGNITIVE AND PERCEPTUAL DEFICIT?

The detailed assessment of cognitive and perceptual deficits is complex and diagnosis requires a comprehensive assessment carried out by a professional with specialist knowledge. This is usually a clinical psychologist or occupational therapist. However, all neurologically impaired patients should be screened for cognitive/perceptual deficit and therefore the inexperienced therapist should be aware of the possible deficits and how they present.

An understanding of the hierarchy of cognition and perception discussed above will facilitate ideas about simple tasks or specific questions that the therapist could implement in order to test each category. For example, to test the concepts of visuospatial perception, the patient could be asked to place a button in a cup, behind a cup, to the right of a cup. For body schema the patient should be able to point out their own and the therapist's shoulder, hand and foot. However, caution is advised as many of these processes rely on many sources of information and interact with each other. The therapist should also account for any motor deficits which may influence the patient's responses.

More severe deficits may be easily discernible, however it may be much harder to identify more subtle problems. The novice therapist should discuss any suspected deficit with a more senior therapist and refer the patient to the relevant professional if the symptom is not being managed.

OUTCOME MEASURES

RESEARCH
As below.

CLINICAL
- Stroop test for selective attention
- Mini Mental State Exam (MMSE)
- Chessington Occupational Therapy Neurological Assessment Battery (COTNAB). Validated for adults with brain injury and stroke
- Rivermead perceptual assessment battery.

REFERENCES AND FURTHER READING

Boyd LA, Winstein CJ: Implicit motor sequence learning in humans following unilateral stroke: the impact of practice and explicit knowledge, *Neuroscience Letters* 298:65–69, 2001.

Broetz D, Karnath H-O: New aspects for the physiotherapy of pushing behaviour, *NeuroRehabilitation* 20:133–138, 2005.

Demakis GJ: The neuropsychology of Parkinson's disease, *Disease-a-Month* 533:152–155, 2007.

Kandel ER, Schwartz JH, Jessell TM: *Principles of neural science*, ed 4, New York, 2000, McGraw-Hill.

Karnath H-O: Pusher syndrome: a frequent but little-known disturbance of body orientation perception, *Journal of Neurology* 254:415–424, 2007.

Multiple Sclerosis Resource Centre: Cognitive problems in MS, 2002, www.msrc.co.uk/printablecfm?pageid=1272.

Parkinson's Disease Society: *The professional's guide to Parkinson's disease*, 2007, www.parkinsons.org.uk/pdf/B126_professionalguidepdf.

Royal College of Physicians: *National Clinical Guidelines for Stroke*, ed 2, Intercollegiate stroke working party, 2004, www.rcp.london.ac.uk.

Shumway-Cook A, Woollacott MH: *Motor control translating research into clinical practice*, ed 3, Philadelphia, 2007, Lippincott Williams and Wilkins.

Falls

WHAT ARE FALLS?

A fall is a descent under the force of gravity and can be a major cause of personal injury. The consequences of a fall may result in a mild soft tissue injury but can also be fatal.

PHYSICAL INJURY

Fracture: In particular the neck of the femur (Hyndman et al. 2002). The incidence of fracture as a result of a fall is between 0.6% and 8.5% (Teasell et al. 2002). In cerebrovascular accident (CVA) the most common fracture is of the hip (45–59%) on the affected side (Dennis et al. 2002).

Soft tissue injuries: Include bruises and open wounds (risk of infection) (Hyndman et al. 2002).

PSYCHOSOCIAL IMPACT

Fear of further falls: Lack of confidence often leads to activity avoidance, greater disability, lack of independence and social isolation (Hyndman et al. 2002; Mackintosh et al. 2005). Activity avoidance also has many secondary consequences which perpetuate the chance of a fall, e.g. reduced exercise tolerance, impaired balance responses, altered body schema, depressed mood and loss of bone mineral density (osteoporosis).

The aim of The National Service Framework for older people (Standard 6 – Falls) (NSF 2001) is to reduce the number of falls which result in serious injury and ensure effective treatment and rehabilitation for those who have fallen. In order to achieve this, preventive intervention and curative rehabilitation are viewed as equally important and therefore an assessment of the relevant risk factors is essential.

RISK FACTORS FOR FALLING

Being aware of the potential risk factors for falls allows the therapist to predict and hopefully prevent a fall. The aetiology of falls is multifactorial with the risk of falling increased with the number of risk factors. There is substantial evidence related to falls in the older person which takes into account the neurological pathologies associated with this age group.

The main points will be drawn out here, however for a more comprehensive understanding of this area the reader is referred to the NSF (2001) and The National Institute for Clinical Excellence guidelines for the assessment and treatment of falls in the older person (NICE 2004). Fall-related risk factors for the elderly are generally classified into intrinsic and extrinsic.

Intrinsic

- Mobility problems: Walking speed, balance (Mackintosh et al. 2006), lower limb muscle strength
- Cognitive factors: Poor attention (Anstey et al. 2006), depression
- Impaired vision: Impaired depth perception strongest risk factor for multiple falls (Lord and Dayhew 2001)
- Taking four or more medications
- Osteoporosis (loss of bone mineral density): Increases the risk of fracture
- Postural hypotension.

Extrinsic: environmental factors

- Hazards: Loose rugs, unsuitable clothing and footwear, steep stairs
- Poor lighting

- Lack of safety equipment (grab rails)
- Time of day: Most falls occur at home during the day (Hyndman et al. 2002; NSF 2001).

PATHOLOGY SPECIFIC RISK FACTORS

Neurologically impaired patients may also have additional pathology specific risk factors. For example:

CVA

- Various motor dysfunctions: (Yates et al. 2002)
- Altered sensation: (Yates et al. 2002; Soyuer and Ozturk 2007)
- Cognitive deficits: (Stapleton et al. 2001; Yates et al. 2002), including attention deficits (Hyndman and Ashburn 2003) and depressed mood (Ugur et al. 2000)
- Impaired balance: (Stapleton et al. 2001; Teasell et al. 2002)
- More dependency in activities of daily living (ADLs): (Lamb et al. 2003; Hyndman et al. 2003)
- Fear of falling after initial fall: (Belgen et al. 2006).

Predictive risk factors for falls in CVA
- Fear of falling – Previous falls: Error in perceived stability limits (Takatori et al. 2009)
- Although altered gait and balance are risk factors for falls they are not accurate in terms of predicting falls (Harris et al. 2005)
- ADLs: Patients who are more dependent are more likely to fall (Teasell 2002).

Parkinson's disease (PD)

- Longer disease duration/an advanced stage of disease (Pickering et al. 2007)
- Postural instability/poor balance (Bloem et al. 2006; Vaugoyeau et al. 2007)
- Difficulty initiating saving reactions (step or upper limb) due to an impairment of anticipatory postural adjustments (King and Horak 2008)
- Mobility:
  - Freezing of gait (Moore et al. 2007)
  - Turning slower and taking more steps than control subjects (Crenna et al. 2007)
  - Axial stiffness resulting in loss of intersegmental coordination (Baltadjieva et al. 2006)
- Altered body schema resulting in an *overestimate* of the limits of stability (Kamata et al. 2007)
- Medication side-effects: Levodopa may cause violent dyskinesias or postural hypotension (Vestergaard et al. 2007)
- Fear of falling after initial fall.

Predictive risk factors of fall in PD

- Previous fallers: Two or more falls in the previous year (Pickering et al. 2007)
- In non-fallers:
  - Fear of falling: (Dennison et al. 2007; Pickering et al. 2007)
  - Number of near misses: (Pickering et al. 2007)
  - Postural hypotension: A decrease of greater than 20–10 mmHg on standing (Williams et al. 2006; Dennison et al. 2007).

Clinical hints and tips

Fear of falling stands out as a high-risk factor for falls and is related to the concept of self-efficacy. That is, an individual's beliefs in his or her ability to perform a given task or behaviour. These beliefs may influence the choice and participation in activities, with low self-efficacy resulting in avoidance. It should be noted that all neurologically impaired patients are potentially at risk of falling and although the above highlights falls in an elderly population, attention to the falls history and associated risk factors for younger patients is also advisable.

WHY DO I NEED TO ASSESS FALLS?

There is a high incidence of falls in neurologically impaired patients resulting in high economic costs and social problems (Lamb et al. 2003; Harris et al. 2005; Belgen et al. 2006). In Parkinson's disease, the fall rate for first time fallers is reported as 21% and for multi-fallers 46% (Pickering et al. 2007), with the likelihood of sustaining a fracture increased twofold (Vestergaard et al. 2007). In CVA, in the community setting, 40–73% patients fall within the first 6 months (Hyndman et al. 2003), with the greatest number falling while walking (39–90%) (Hyndman et al. 2002). In the inpatient setting, 14–39% of patients fall (Suzuki et al. 2005; Teasell et al. 2002; Langhorne et al. 2000), with the greatest number falling during transfers (Suzuki et al. 2005).

HOW DO I ASSESS FALLS?

The NICE (2004) guideline on falls in the older person (>65 years old) recommends that all patients within this criteria be asked routinely whether they have fallen in the past year and then about the frequency, context and characteristics of the fall(s). When the individual reports recurrent falls within the year, the NICE guidance is that they should be offered a multifactorial falls risk assessment which involves a multidisciplinary team approach.

1. Identification of falls history
2. Assessment of gait, balance and mobility, and muscle weakness
3. Assessment of osteoporosis risk
4. Assessment of the older person's perceived functional ability and fear relating to falling
5. Assessment of visual impairment
6. Assessment of cognitive impairment and neurological examination
7. Assessment of urinary incontinence
8. Assessment of home hazards
9. Cardiovascular examination and medication review.

The therapist will be involved in providing information for several of these aspects. First, the initial enquiry of 'have you fallen in the last year?', with follow-up questioning to ascertain more detailed information related to the falls history. Second, elements of the objective assessment will be valuable to the multifactorial risk assessment, functional assessment (S3.18), gait (S3.19), balance (S3.32), muscle strength (S3.30) and muscle tone (S3.21).

RECORDING

In the subjective section of the assessment, a section dedicated to falls is advisable to record the initial enquiry and relevant falls history.

ANALYSIS

Following assessment of any relevant risk factors for falls, the therapist must communicate with the patient's key worker or whoever is coordinating the multifactorial assessment. Only with all the relevant information can the team identify individuals who are at high risk of falling and implement an appropriate multidisciplinary and multiagency intervention. The Cochrane Library reviews (Cameron et al. 2005; Gillespie et al. 2009) make recommendations for best practice in terms of falls management.

Even if the reported falls history does not warrant a full multifactorial assessment a discussion with the patient offering education and advice related to falls and any potential risk factors may still be advisable.

OUTCOME MEASURES

RESEARCH
As below.

CLINICAL
Commonly used outcome measures for falls risk assessment in relation to balance and gait are the Timed up and go test; Turn 180 degrees; Performance-oriented assessment of mobility problems (Tinetti scale); Functional reach; Dynamic gait index; Berg balance scale. However, it is unclear which tool or assessment instrument is the most predictive of future falls (NICE 2004).

As fear of falling is identified as a predictive risk factor and a consequence of a fall, its consideration by all involved with the patient's care is advised. Two recommended scales are the Activities-specific Balance Confidence (ABC) scale and the Falls Efficacy Scale (Peretz et al. 2006). However, the NICE guidelines (2004) state that simply asking the patient 'if they are fearful of falling?' may be as useful as carrying out complex measures.

REFERENCES
Anstey KJ, von Sanden C, Luszcz MA: An 8-year prospective study of the relationship between cognitive performance and falling in very old adults, *Journal of American Geriatrics Society* 54:1169–1176, 2006.

Baltadjieva R, Giladi N, Gruendlinger L, et al: Marked alterations in the gait timing and rhythmicity of patients with de novo Parkinson's disease, *European Journal of Neuroscience* 24:1815–1820, 2006.

Belgen B, Beninato M, Sullivan PE, et al: The association of balance capacity and falls self-efficacy with history of falling in community-dwelling people with chronic stroke, *Archives of Physical Medicine and Rehabilitation* 87:554–561, 2006.

Bloem BR, Grimbergen YA, van Dijk JG, et al: The 'posture second' strategy: a review of wrong priorities in Parkinson's disease, *Journal of Neurological Sciences* 248:196–204, 2006.

Cameron ID, Murray GR, Gillespie LD, et al: Interventions for preventing falls in older people in residential care facilities and hospitals, Cochrane Database of Systematic Reviews 2005 Issue 3. CD005465, 2005.

Crenna P, Carpinella I, Rabuffetti M, et al: The association between impaired turning and normal straight walking in Parkinson's disease, *Gait Posture* 26:172–178, 2007.

Dennis MS, Lo KM, McDowall M, et al: Fractures after stroke: frequency types and associations, *Stroke* 333:728–734, 2002.

Dennison AC, Noorigian JV, Robinson KM, et al: Falling in Parkinson disease: identifying and prioritizing risk factors in recurrent fallers, *American Journal of Physical Medicine and Rehabilitation* 86:621–632, 2007.

Gillespie LD, Robertson MC, Gillespie WJ, et al: Interventions for preventing falls in older people living in the community, Cochrane Database of Systematic Reviews Issue 2. CD007146, 2009.

Harris JE, Eng JJ, Marigold DS, et al: Relationship of balance and mobility to fall incidence in people with chronic stroke, *Physical therapy* 852:150–158, 2005.

Hyndman D, Ashburn A: People with stroke living in the community: attention deficits balance ADL ability and falls, *Disability and Rehabilitation* 25:817–822, 2003.

Hyndman D, Ashburn A, Stack E: Fall events among people with stroke living in the community: circumstances of falls and characteristics of fallers, *Archives of Physical Medicine and Rehabilitation* 83:165–170, 2002.

Kamata N, Matsuo Y, Yoneda T, et al: Overestimation of stability limits leads to a high frequency of falls in patients with Parkinson's disease, *Clinical Rehabilitation* 21:357–361, 2007.

King L, Horak FB: Lateral stepping for postural correction in Parkinson's disease, *Archives of Physical Medicine and Rehabilitation* 89:492–499, 2008.

Lamb SE, Ferrucci L, Volapto S, et al: Women's Health and Aging Study Risk factors for falling in home-dwelling older women with stroke: The Women's Health and Aging Study, *Stroke* 342:494–501, 2003.

Langhorne P, Stott DJ, Robertson L, et al: Medical complications after stroke, *Stroke* 31:1223–1229, 2000.

Lord SR, Dayhew J: Visual risk factors for falls, *Journal of American Geriatric Society* 49:508–515, 2001.

Mackintosh SF, Hill K, Dodd KJ, et al: Falls and injury prevention should be part of every stroke rehabilitation plan, *Clinical Rehabilitation* 194:441–451, 2005.

Mackintosh SF, Hill KD, Dodd KJ, et al: Balance score and a history of falls in hospital predict recurrent falls in the 6 months following stroke rehabilitation, *Archives of Physical Medicine and Rehabilitation* 87:1583–1589, 2006.

Moore O, Peretz C, Giladi N: Freezing of gait affects quality of life of people with Parkinson's disease beyond its relationships with mobility and gait, *Movement Disorders* 22:2192–2195, 2007.

NICE: *National Institute for Clinical Excellence guidelines for the assessment and treatment of falls in the older person,* 2004, www.nice.org.uk/nicemedia/pdf/CG021fullguidelinepdf.

NSF: *National Service Framework for older people, Standard 6,* 2001, www.dhgov.uk/prod_consum_dh/groups/dh_digitalassets/@dh/@en/documents/digitalasset/dh_4071283pdf.

Peretz C, Herman T, Hausdorff JM, et al: Assessing fear of falling: can a short version of the activities-specific balance confidence scale be useful? *Movement Disorders* 21:2101–2105, 2006.

Pickering RM, Grimbergen YA, Rigney U, et al: A meta-analysis of six prospective studies of falling in Parkinson's disease, *Movement Disorders* 22:1892–1900, 2007.

Soyuer F, Ozturk A: The effect of spasticity sense and walking aids in falls of people after chronic stroke, *Disability Rehabilitation* 299:679–687, 2007.

Stapleton T, Ashburn A, Stack E: A pilot study of attention deficits balance control and falls in the subacute stage following stroke, *Clinical Rehabilitation* 154:437–444, 2001.

Suzuki T, Sonoda S, Misawa K: Incidence and consequence of falls in inpatient rehabilitation of stroke patients, *Experimental Aging Research* 31:457–469, 2005.

Takatori K, Okada Y, Shomoto K, et al: Does assessing error in perceiving postural limits by testing functional reach predict likelihood of falls in hospitalized stroke patients? *Clinical Rehabilitation* 23:568–575, 2009.

Teasell R, McRae M, Foley N, et al: The incidence and consequences of falls in stroke patients during inpatient rehabilitation: factors associated with high risk, *Archives of Physical Medicine and Rehabilitation* 833:329–333, 2002.

Ugur C, Gucuyener D, Uzuner N, et al: Characteristics of falling in patients with stroke, *Journal of Neurology Neurosurgery and Psychiatry* 69:649–651, 2000.

Vaugoyeau M, Viel S, Assaiante C, et al: Impaired vertical postural control and proprioceptive integration deficits in Parkinson's disease, *Neuroscience* 146:852–863, 2007.

Vestergaard P, Rejnmark L, Mosekilde L: Fracture risk associated with parkinsonism and anti-Parkinson drugs, *Calcified Tissue International* 81:153–161, 2007.

Williams DR, Watt HC, Lees AJ: Predictors of falls and fractures in bradykinetic rigid syndromes: a retrospective study, *Journal of Neurology Neurosurgery and Psychiatry* 77:468–473, 2006.

Yates JS, Lai SM, Duncan PW, et al: Falls in community dwelling stroke survivors: an accumulated impairments model, *Journal of Rehabilitation Research and Development* 385–394, 2002.

Index